T0176160

Hemophilia and Hemostasis

Hemophilia and Hemostasis

A Case-Based Approach to Management

EDITED BY

Alice D. Ma, MD
Associate Professor of Medicine
Division of Hematology/Oncology
University of North Carolina
Chapel Hill, NC, USA

Harold R. Roberts, MD
Emeritus Professor of Medicine and Pathology
Division of Hematology/Oncology
University of North Carolina
Chapel Hill, NC, USA

Miguel A. Escobar, MD
Associate Professor of Medicine and Pediatrics
Division of Hematology
University of Texas Health Science Center at Houston
Director, Gulf States Hemophilia and Thrombophilia Center
Houston, TX, USA

SECOND EDITION

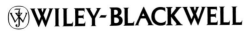

WILEY-BLACKWELL

A John Wiley & Sons, Ltd., Publication

This edition first published 2013, © 2007, 2013 by John Wiley & Sons Limited.

Wiley-Blackwell is an imprint of John Wiley & Sons, formed by the merger of Wiley's global Scientific, Technical and Medical business with Blackwell Publishing.

Registered Office: John Wiley & Sons, Ltd, The Atrium, Southern Gate, Chichester, West Sussex, PO19 8SQ, UK

Editorial Offices: 9600 Garsington Road, Oxford, OX4 2DQ, UK

The Atrium, Southern Gate, Chichester, West Sussex, PO19 8SQ, UK

111 River Street, Hoboken, NJ 07030-5774, USA

For details of our global editorial offices, for customer services and for information about how to apply for permission to reuse the copyright material in this book please see our website at www.wiley.com/wiley-blackwell

The right of the author to be identified as the author of this work has been asserted in accordance with the UK Copyright, Designs and Patents Act 1988.

All rights reserved. No part of this publication may be reproduced, stored in a retrieval system, or transmitted, in any form or by any means, electronic, mechanical, photocopying, recording or otherwise, except as permitted by the UK Copyright, Designs and Patents Act 1988, without the prior permission of the publisher.

Designations used by companies to distinguish their products are often claimed as trademarks. All brand names and product names used in this book are trade names, service marks, trademarks or registered trademarks of their respective owners. The publisher is not associated with any product or vendor mentioned in this book. This publication is designed to provide accurate and authoritative information in regard to the subject matter covered. It is sold on the understanding that the publisher is not engaged in rendering professional services. If professional advice or other expert assistance is required, the services of a competent professional should be sought.

The contents of this work are intended to further general scientific research, understanding, and discussion only and are not intended and should not be relied upon as recommending or promoting a specific method, diagnosis, or treatment by physicians for any particular patient. The publisher and the author make no representations or warranties with respect to the accuracy or completeness of the contents of this work and specifically disclaim all warranties, including without limitation any implied warranties of fitness for a particular purpose. In view of ongoing research, equipment modifications, changes in governmental regulations, and the constant flow of information relating to the use of medicines, equipment, and devices, the reader is urged to review and evaluate the information provided in the package insert or instructions for each medicine, equipment, or device for, among other things, any changes in the instructions or indication of usage and for added warnings and precautions. Readers should consult with a specialist where appropriate. The fact that an organization or Website is referred to in this work as a citation and/or a potential source of further information does not mean that the author or the publisher endorses the information the organization or Website may provide or recommendations it may make. Further, readers should be aware that Internet Websites listed in this work may have changed or disappeared between when this work was written and when it is read. No warranty may be created or extended by any promotional statements for this work. Neither the publisher nor the author shall be liable for any damages arising herefrom.

Library of Congress Cataloging-in-Publication Data

Hemophilia and hemostasis : a case-based approach to management / edited by Alice D. Ma, Harold R. Roberts, Miguel A. Escobar. – 2nd ed.
    p. ; cm.
  Rev. ed. of: Haemophilia and haemostasis. c2007.
  Includes bibliographical references and index.
  ISBN 978-0-470-65976-2 (hardback : alk. paper)
  I. Ma, Alice. II. Roberts, H. R. (Harold Ross) III. Escobar, Miguel A. IV. Haemophilia and haemostasis.
  [DNLM: 1. Blood Coagulation Disorders, Inherited–therapy–Case Reports. 2. Thrombosis–therapy–Case Reports. WH 322]
  616.1'572–dc23

2012017384

A catalogue record for this book is available from the British Library.

Wiley also publishes its books in a variety of electronic formats. Some content that appears in print may not be available in electronic books.

Set in 9.5/13pt Meridien by SPi Publisher Services, Pondicherry, India
Printed and bound in Singapore by Markono Print Media Pte Ltd

1   2013

Contents

Contributors

Anas Alrwas, MD
Resident, Internal Medicine
University of Texas Health Science Center
at Houston
Houston, TX, USA

Tyler Buckner, MD
Hematology Fellow
Pediatric Hematology/Oncology
Adult Hematology
University of North Carolina School
of Medicine
Chapel Hill, NC, USA

Benjamin Carcamo, MD
Clinical Assistant Professor
Pediatric Hematology Oncology
Providence Memorial Hospital
Texas Tech University, School of Medicine
El Paso, TX, USA

Miguel A. Escobar, MD
Associate Professor of Medicine and Pediatrics
Division of Hematology
University of Texas Health Science Center
at Houston
Director, Gulf States Hemophilia and
Thrombophilia Center
Houston, TX, USA

Matthew Foster, MD
Assistant Professor of Medicine
Division of Hematology/Oncology
University of North Carolina School
of Medicine
Chapel Hill, NC, USA

Raj Sundar Kasthuri, MD
Assistant Professor of Medicine
Division of Hematology/Oncology
University of North Carolina School
of Medicine
Chapel Hill, NC, USA

Kristy Lee, MS, CGC
Clinical Assistant Professor
Department of Genetics
University of North Carolina School of Medicine
Chapel Hill, NC, USA

Alice D. Ma, MD
Associate Professor of Medicine
Division of Hematology/Oncology
University of North Carolina School
of Medicine
Chapel Hill, NC, USA

Marshall Mazepa, MD
Senior Fellow
Division of Hematology/Oncology
University of North Carolina School
of Medicine
Chapel Hill, NC, USA

Trinh T. Nguyen, DO
Assistant Professor of Pediatrics
Division of Hematology
University of Texas Health Science Center
at Houston
Gulf States Hemophilia and Thrombophilia
Center
Houston, TX, USA

Nidra Rodriguez, MD
Assistant Professor of Pediatrics
Division of Hematology
The University of Texas Health Science Center
at Houston
MD Anderson Cancer Center
Gulf States Hemophilia & Thrombophilia Center
Houston, TX, USA

**E. Carlos Rodriguez-Merchan,
MD, PhD**
Consultant Orthopaedic Surgeon and Associate
Professor of Orthopaedics
La Paz University Hospital
Universidad Autonoma
Madrid, Spain

Jenny M. Splawn, PharmD
Providence Memorial Hospital
El Paso, TX, USA

Tzu-Fei Wang, MD
Fellow
Divisions of Hematology and Oncology
Washington University School of Medicine
Saint Louis, MO, USA

Foreword

I am delighted to respond to the invitation to provide a brief introduction to the second edition of *Hemophilia and Hemostasis: A Case-Based Approach to Management*. The popularity of this text stems from its unique case-based approach. Drs Roberts, Ma, and Escobar are renowned and frequently consulted experts in the management of patients with bleeding disorders. Although the hemophilias and other inherited bleeding disorders have been the focus of a comparatively large body of literature, there are remarkably few randomized-controlled clinical trials on which to base firm evidence-based recommendations. This fact was most recently brought home to me as a member of the team charged with revising the World Federation of Hemophilia's *Treatment Guidelines*; our goal was to provide appropriately graded recommendations of the literature and generally accepted practices for the practicing clinician. Unfortunately, the paucity of high-quality level 1 evidence does not obviate the need to make clinical decisions on a daily basis when caring for patients with bleeding disorders. The authors address these management dilemmas in a comprehensive series of "mini-chapters" that provide an easy reference format for the reader. In this day and age of electronic fingertip access to state-of-the-art reviews on PubMed, it is sometimes said that textbooks are obsolete before they are even published. While there may be some truth to this viewpoint in the case of standard texts, no amount of electronic searching can provide the ready access to the august consensus opinions of these seasoned experts, who have "been down that same road" before. As such, this book is a must for every hematologist or nurse who is charged with taking care of patients with bleeding disorders.

Nigel S. Key MB ChB FRCP
Harold R. Roberts Distinguished Professor of Medicine
and Pathology and Laboratory Medicine
Chief, Section of Hematology
Director, UNC Hemophilia and Thrombosis Center
Chapel Hill, NC

PART I

Hemophilia A and Hemophilia B

SECTION I
General Overview

The Hemophilic Ankle: An Update

E. Carlos Rodriguez-Merchan

La Paz University Hospital and Universidad Autonoma, Madrid, Spain

Q	What is the latest information regarding the treatment of hemophilic arthropathy in the ankle?

It is well known that the ankles in hemophilic patients tend to bleed, beginning at an early age of 2–5 years. The synovium is only able to reabsorb a small amount of intra-articular blood; if the amount of blood is excessive, the synovium will hypertrophy as a compensating mechanism, so that eventually the affected joint will show an increase in size of the synovium, leading to hypertrophic chronic hemophilic synovitis. The hypertrophic synovium is very richly vascularized, so that small injuries will easily make the joint rebleed. The final result will be the vicious cycle of hemarthrosis–synovitis–hemarthrosis, which eventually will result in hemophilic arthropathy (Figure I1.1).

Pathogenesis of synovitis and cartilage damage in hemophilia: experimental studies

Hooiveld *et al.* (2004) investigated the effect of a limited number of joint bleedings, combined with loading of the affected joint, in the development of progressive degenerative joint damage. They concluded that experimental joint bleedings, when combined with loading (weight-bearing) of the involved joint, result in features of progressive degenerative joint damage, whereas similar joint hemorrhages without joint loading do not. The authors suggest that this might reflect a possible mechanism of joint damage in hemophilia. In two other papers (Hakobyan *et al.* 2004;

Hemophilia and Hemostasis: A Case-Based Approach to Management, Second Edition.
Edited by Alice D. Ma, Harold R. Roberts, Miguel A. Escobar.
© 2013 John Wiley & Sons, Ltd. Published 2013 by John Wiley & Sons, Ltd.

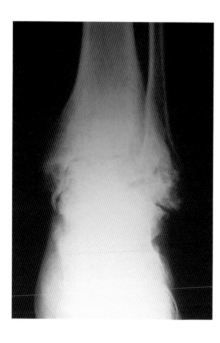

Figure I1.1 Severe hemophilic arthropathy of the ankle in an adult hemophilia patient.

Valentino *et al.* 2004), hemophilic arthropathy was studied in animal models. Despite these interesting papers, the pathogenesis of hemophilic arthropathy remains poorly understood.

The best way to protect against hemophilic arthropathy (cartilage damage) is primary prophylaxis beginning at a very early age. Starting prophylaxis gradually with once-weekly injections has the presumed advantage of avoiding the use of a central venous access device, such as a PortaCath, which is otherwise often necessary for frequent injections in very young boys. The decision to institute early full prophylaxis by means of a port has to be balanced against the child's bleeding tendency, the family's social situation, and the experience of the specific hemophilia center. The reported complication rates for infection and thrombosis have varied considerably from center to center. Risk of infection can be reduced by repeated education of patients and staff, effective surveillance routines and limitations on the number of individuals allowed to use the device. In discussing options for early therapy, the risks and benefits should be thoroughly discussed with the parents. For children with inhibitors needing daily infusions for immune tolerance induction, a central venous line is often unavoidable and is associated with an increased incidence of infections.

From a practical point of view, radiosynovectomy, together with primary prophylaxis to avoid joint bleeding, can help to halt hemophilic synovitis. Ideally, however, radiosynovectomy should be performed before the articular cartilage has eroded. Radiosynovectomy is a relatively simple, virtually painless, and inexpensive treatment for chronic hemophilic

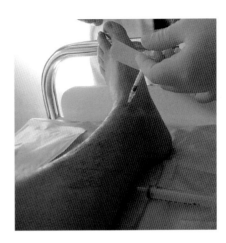

Figure I1.2 Radiosynovectomy of the ankle with 186 rhenium.

synovitis, even in patients with inhibitors, and is the best choice for patients with persistent synovitis.

Radiosynovectomy

Radiosynovectomy is the intra-articular injection of a radioactive material to diminish the degree of synovial hypertrophy and to decrease the number and frequency of hemarthroses (Figure I1.2). Radioactive substances have been used for the treatment of chronic hemophilic synovitis for many years. Radiation causes fibrosis within the subsynovial connective tissue of the joint capsule and synovium. It also affects the complex vascular system, in that some vessels become obstructed; however, articular cartilage is not affected by radiation.

The indication for radiosynovectomy is chronic hemophilic synovitis causing recurrent hemarthroses, unresponsive to treatment. There are three basic types of synovectomies: chemical synovectomy, radiosynovectomy, and arthroscopic synovectomy. On average, the efficacy of the procedure ranges from 76 to 80%, and can be performed at any age. The procedure slows the cartilaginous damage which intra-articular blood tends to produce in the long term.

Radiosynovectomy (Yttrium-90, Phosphorus-32, and Rhenium-186) can be repeated up to three times at 6-month intervals. Chemical synovectomy can be repeated weekly up to 10–15 times if rifampicin is used. After 35 years of using radiosynovectomy world wide, no damage has been reported in relation to the radioactive materials. Radiosynovectomy is currently the preferred procedure when radioactive materials are available; however, rifampicin is an effective alternative method if radioactive materials are not available. Several joints can be injected in a single session, but it is best to limit injections to two joints at the same time.

There are two interesting papers that focus on the treatment of chronic hemophilic synovitis. Corrigan *et al.* (2003) have used oral D-penicillamine for the treatment of 16 patients. The drug was given as a single dose in the morning before breakfast. The dose was 5–10 mg/kg bodyweight, not to exceed 10 mg/kg in children, or 750 mg/day in adults. The duration of treatment was 2 months to 1 year (median 3 months). Ten patients had an unequivocal response, 3 had a reduction in palpable synovium and 3 had no response. Minor reversible drug side effects occurred in 2 patients (proteinuria in one and a rash in the other).

Radossi *et al.* (2003) have used intra-articular injections of rifamycin. Among a large cohort of nearly 500 patients, they treated 28 patients during a 2-year period. The patients followed an on-demand replacement therapy program and developed single or multiple joint chronic synovitis. The indications for chemical synovectomy were symptoms of chronic synovitis referred by patients reported in a questionnaire. In Radossi's series there were 5 patients with inhibitors to factor VIII. Their average age was 34 years. Rifamycin (250 mg) was diluted in 10 mL of saline solution and 1–5 mL was then injected into the joint. The follow-up ranged from 6 to 24 months. Thirty-five joints were treated with 169 infiltrations in total. Rifamycin was injected once a week for 5 weeks, i.e. the patient had to come to hospital at weekly intervals. Twenty-four procedures were considered effective in 19 patients according to the evaluation scale, while 6 treatments were considered fair to poor. Five patients (six joints) with anti-factor VIII inhibitors were treated. In four joints the results were good, while in the two remaining joints the results were poor.

There are two main limitations for the use of antibiotics in synovectomy: the procedure is painful, and it should be repeated weekly for many weeks to be effective. In fact, Radossi's schedule included injection of rifamycin into the joints once a week for 5 weeks (Radossi *et al.* 2003). However, they make no mention of the pain associated with the injections. They also state that rifamycin may be indicated when radiosynovectomy is not available, contraindicated for medical reasons, or not accepted by patients. To the best of my knowledge I do not know of any medical contraindications to radiosynovectomy, or why patients should reject such an efficient and safe procedure. The Italian authors state that, to date, they cannot say if their program is able to delay long-term functional impairment because of the lack of a longer follow-up. However, according to their preliminary experience, they consider that rifamycin synovectomy appears to be effective in reducing joint pain and in improving the range of motion.

The study of Corrigan *et al.* (2003), which used D-penicillamine, has two main limitations: the small number of patients and the lack of use of ultrasound and/or magnetic resonance imaging (MRI) for diagnostic purposes. It is also important to emphasize two potential side effects of D-penicillamine: aplastic anemia and renal disease. To minimize the possibility of side effects, Corrigan *et al.* (2003) have suggested that the drug be used on a short-term basis (i.e. 3–6 months) and the amount be restricted (see reference for dosing).

I agree with the authors' statement that radiosynovectomy using intra-articular 90-Yttrium, 32-Phosporus, or 186-Rhenium has been reported to be effective. However, I disagree with the authors' comment that this is an invasive procedure whose long-term safety has not been established. In fact, the long-term safety has been established after 35 years of using radiosynovectomy world wide, with no damage reported in relation to the radioactive materials (Hakobyan *et al.* 2004).

It is important to emphasize that controversy exists regarding which type of synovectomy is better. Most authors in developed countries use radiosynovectomy (186-Rhenium, 90-Yttrium, 32-Phosphorus), while others utilize chemical synovectomy mainly because of the lack of availability of radioactive materials. My view is that further studies with an adequate number of patients and an appropriate follow-up are needed to confirm the efficacy of oral penicillamine and rifamycin synovectomy for chronic hemophilic synovitis. In other words, the aforementioned papers are preliminary studies requiring confirmation. Meanwhile, the general recommendation is to use 186-Rhenium, 90-Yttrium, or 32-Phosporus radiosynovectomy, because these agents have proved to be efficient for the treatment of chronic hemophilic synovitis, even in patients with inhibitors.

Hemophilic arthropathy of the ankle and subtalar joints

Chang *et al.* (2001) have analyzed podiatric surgery in hemophilic arthropathy of the ankle and subtalar joints. This condition often results in severe pain and physical limitations. Conservative treatment (splints, braces, wedge insoles, and calipers) should always be attempted prior to surgery. The most common surgical approaches are arthroscopic synovectomy, arthroscopic débridement (Figure I1.3), arthroplasty and arthrodesis (Figure I1.4). Finally, the authors describe an interesting case of avascular necrosis of the talus, ankle/joint degeneration with periarticular osseous fragmentation, a cyst in the medial aspect of the talar dome and a fracture of the os trigonum with resultant hypertrophy of soft tissues.

The most common deformities affecting the ankle and subtalar joints are fixed plantar flexion due to degeneration of the anterior part of the

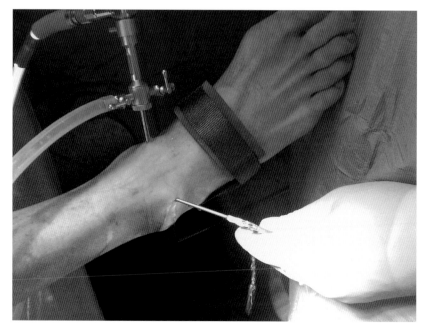

Figure I1.3 Arthroscopy of the ankle for arthroscopic synovectomy and arthroscopic débridement.

ankle, varus hindfoot due to malalignment of the subtalar joint, and valgus rotation of the ankle due to differential overgrowth of the distal tibial epiphysis during adolescence or progressive arthropathy during maturity. The process always starts with a single or recurrent hemarthrosis, which is extremely painful and results in an equinus or plantar flexion position of the ankle. This deformity, initially correctable, eventually becomes fixed.

Probably the first treatment to be considered for recurrent ankle hemarthroses is radiosynovectomy. Another common procedure to prevent fixed equinus deformity is lengthening of the Achilles tendon. Sometimes a large osteophyte develops on the anterior part of the ankle which can cause severe pain (Figure I1.5). Surgical removal of the osteophyte (queilectomy) is sometimes indicated. When the ankle joint shows an important degree of malalignment, a supramalleolar valgus or varus osteotomy is indicated.

In advanced hemophilic arthropathy, an ankle arthrodesis or arthroplasty should be considered. The main indications for these are intractable pain not relieved by alternative treatments, and severe deformity. Regular prophylactic transfusions of clotting factor may prevent recurrent bleeds and further development of hemarthrosis. Ankle arthrodesis has been associated with better long-term results than ankle arthroplasty (rarely performed in hemophilia today). [For a more detailed description of ankle

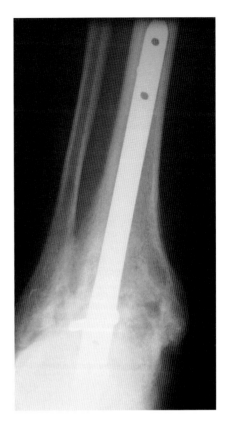

Figure I1.4 Ankle arthrodesis with a retrograde locked intramedullary nail in the same patient of Figure I1.1.

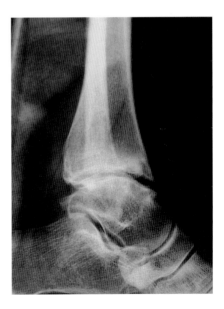

Figure I1.5 Anterior ostephyte of the ankle in a hemophilia patient.

hemarthropathy, the reader is referred to the original submission by Dr. Rodriguez-Merchan. www.haemostasis-forum.org.]

Rehabilitation and physiotherapy

The importance of pre-operative and post-operative rehabilitation of the ankle joint in hemophilia must be emphasized. Children must utilize the resources available and seek early consultation with their center's rehabilitation physician and physiotherapist. Using the techniques available, rehabilitation has been shown to speed recovery, reduce pain, and prevent contractures. Physiotherapy is important to ankle rehabilitation of patients following surgical procedures and the physical therapist must work closely with the orthopedic surgeon.

Conclusions

Radiosynovectomy is a very effective procedure that decreases both the frequency and the intensity of recurrent intra-articular bleeds related to joint synovitis. The procedure should be performed as soon as possible to minimize the degree of articular cartilage damage. It can also be used in patients with inhibitors with minimal risk of complications.

Radiosynovectomy is the best choice for patients with persistent synovitis. Personal experience and the general recommendation among orthopedic surgeons and hematologists is that when three early consecutive radiosynovectomies (repeated every 3 months) fail to halt synovitis, an arthroscopic synovectomy should be immediately considered. For advanced hemophilic arthropathy of the ankle, the best solution is an ankle arthrodesis. (For further details on the issues in this article, the reader is referred to the Further Reading section below, in which the items are given in chronological order.)

References

Chang TJ, Mohamed S, Hambleton J. (2001) Hemophilic arthropathy: considerations in management. *J Am Podiatr Med Assoc* **91**: 406–414.

Corrigan JJ, Jr., Damiano ML, Leissinger C, Wulff K. (2003) Treatment of chronic haemophilic synovitis in humans with D-penicillamine. *Haemophilia* **9**: 64–68.

Gamble JG, Bellah J, Rinsky LA, Glader B. (1991) Arthropathy of the ankle in hemophilia. *J Bone Joint Surg Am* **73**: 1008–1015.

Hakobyan N, Kazarian T, Jabbar AA, *et al.* (2004) Pathobiology of hemophilic synovitis I: overexpression of md m2 oncogene. *Blood* **104**: 2060–2064.

Hooiveld MJ, Roosendaal G, Jacobs KM, *et al.* (2004) Initiation of degenerative joint damage by experimental bleeding combined with loading of the joint: a possible mechanism of hemophilic arthropathy. *Arthritis Rheum* **50**: 2024–2031.

Lofqvist T, Petersson C, Nilsson IM (1997) Radioactive synoviorthesis in patients with hemophilia with factor inhibitor. *Clin Orthop Relat Res* **343**: 37–41.

Luck J, Lin J, Kasper C, Logan L (2001) Orthopaedic management of hemophilic arthropathy. In: Chapman M (ed.), *Chapman's Orthopaedic Surgery* (3rd edn.). Philadelphia, PA: Lippincott Williams & Wilkins.

Panotopoulos J, Hanslik-Schnabel B, Wanivenhaus A, Trieb K (2005) Outcome of surgical concepts in haemophilic arthropathy of the hindfoot. *Haemophilia* **11**: 468–471.

Radossi P, Baggio R, Petris U, *et al.* (2003) Intra-articular rifamycin in haemophilic arthropathy. *Haemophilia* **9**: 60–63.

Valentino LA, Hakobyan N, Kazarian T, *et al.* (2004) Experimental haemophilic synovitis: rationale and development of a murine model of human factor VIII deficiency. *Haemophilia* **10**: 280–287.

Further reading

Rodriguez-Merchan EC (2006) The haemophilic ankle. *Haemophilia* **12**: 337–344.

Wallny T, Brackmann H, Kraft C, *et al.* (2006) Achilles tendon lengthening for ankle equinus deformity in hemophiliacs: 23 patients followed for 1–24 years. *Acta Orthop* **77**: 164–168.

van der Heide HJ, Nováková I, de Waal Malefijt MC (2006) The feasibility of total ankle prosthesis for severe arthropathy in haemophilia and prothrombin deficiency. *Haemophilia* **12**: 679–682.

Kotwal RS, Acharya A, O'Doherty D (2007) Anterior tibial artery pseudoaneurysm in a patient with hemophilia: a complication of ankle arthroscopy. *J Foot Ankle Surg* **46**: 314–316.

Rodriguez-Merchan EC (2008) Ankle surgery in haemophilia with special emphasis on arthroscopic debridement. *Haemophilia* **14**: 913–919.

Pasta G, Forsyth A, Merchan CR, *et al.* (2008) Orthopaedic management of haemophilia arthropathy of the ankle. *Haemophilia* **14** (Suppl 3): 170–176.

Mann HA, Biring GS, Choudhury MZ, *et al.* (2009) Ankle arthropathy in the haemophilic patient: a description of a novel ankle arthrodesis technique. *Haemophilia* **15**: 458–463.

Barg A, Elsner A, Hefti D, Hintermann B (2010) Haemophilic arthropathy of the ankle treated by total ankle replacement: a case series. *Haemophilia* **16**: 647–655.

Kong M, Kang JO, Choi J, Park SH (2010) A long term result of external beam radiation therapy in hemophilic arthropathy of the ankle in children. *J Korean Med Sci* **25**: 1742–1747.

Tsailas PG, Wiedel JD (2010) Arthrodesis of the ankle and subtalar joints in patients with haemophilic arthropathy. *Haemophilia* **16**: 822–831.

Lobet S, Hermans C, Pasta G, Detrembleur C (2011) Body structure versus body function in haemophilia: the case of haemophilic ankle arthropathy. *Haemophilia* **17**: 508–515.

INTRODUCTION 2

The Hemophilic Knee: An Update

E. Carlos Rodriguez-Merchan

La Paz University Hospital and Universidad Autonoma, Madrid, Spain

Q	What is the latest information regarding the treatment of the hemophilic arthropathy in the knee?

Primary prophylaxis is paramount as a way of preventing the occurrence of hemarthrosis and thereby the onset of hemophilic arthropathy provided that it is started very early in life (Rodriguez-Merchan *et al.* 2011a; Jiminez-Yuste *et al.* 2011). It is well known that the knees of hemophilics tend to bleed from an early age of 2–5 years. The synovial membrane is only able to reabsorb a small amount of intra-articular blood; if the amount of blood is excessive, the synovial membrane will hypertrophy as a compensating mechanism, so that eventually the affected joint will show an increase in size of the synovial membrane – the so-called hypertrophic chronic hemophilic synovitis (Figure I2.1). The hypertrophic synovial membrane is very richly vascularized, so that small injuries will easily make the joint rebleed. The final result will be the classic vicious cycle of hemarthrosis–synovitis–hemarthrosis (Valentino 2010). In this article I will review the most important current therapeutic modalities for the hemophilic knee.

Joint aspiration (arthrocentesis)

The diagnosis and treatment of knee-bleeding episodes must be delivered as early as possible. Additionally, hematological treatment should ideally be administered intensively (enhanced on-demand treatment) until the

Hemophilia and Hemostasis: A Case-Based Approach to Management, Second Edition.
Edited by Alice D. Ma, Harold R. Roberts, Miguel A. Escobar.
© 2013 John Wiley & Sons, Ltd. Published 2013 by John Wiley & Sons, Ltd.

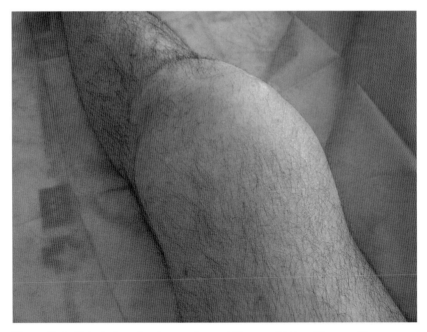

Figure I2.1 Clinical view of an intense hemophilic synovitis in a 23-year-old hemophilia patient previously treated on demand.

resolution of symptoms. Joint aspiration (arthrocentesis) plays an important role in acute and profuse hemarthroses as the presence of blood in the joint leads to chondrocyte apoptosis and chronic synovitis, which will eventually result in joint degeneration (hemophilic arthropathy). Ultrasonography (US) is an appropriate diagnostic technique to assess the evolution of acute hemarthrosis in hemophilia, although MRI remains the gold standard as far as imaging techniques are concerned. A joint aspiration of the knee is a very efficient procedure that can usually be carried out at the outpatient clinic or at the patient's bedside (Jiminez-Yuste *et al.* 2011). Articular punctures must be used in hemophilia for the evacuation of knee voluminous hemarthroses, always under appropriate clotting factor coverage.

Radiosynovectomy
Radiosynovectomy consists of destruction of synovial tissue by intra-articular injection of a radioactive agent. Radioactive substances have been used for the treatment of chronic hemophilic synovitis of the knee for many years (Rodriguez-Merchan 2010, 2007a; Rodriguez-Merchan *et al.* 2007a; De la Corte-Rodriguez *et al.* 2011a, 2011b, 2011c). Radiation causes fibrosis within the subsynovial connective tissue of the joint capsule and synovial membrane. It also affects the complex vascular system, in that some vessels become obstructed; however, articular cartilage is not affected

by radiation. Radioactive substances, therefore, have a radionecrotic effect. The indication for a radiosynovectomy is chronic hemophilic synovitis causing recurrent hemarthroses. On average, the efficacy of radiosynovectomy ranges from 75 to 80%, and can be performed at any age. The procedure slows the cartilaginous damage which intra-articular blood tends to produce in the long term. Radiosynovectomy can be repeated up to three times with 6-month intervals if radioactive materials are used (Yttrium-90, Phosphorus-32, and Rhenium-186), always under factor coverage. After 40 years of using radiation synovectomy world wide, no damage has been reported in relation to the radioactive materials.

Rehabilitation and physiotherapy

The importance of pre-operative and post-operative rehabilitation of the knee joint in hemophilia must be emphasized. Children must utilize the resources available and seek early consultation with their center rehabilitation physician and/or physiotherapist. Using the techniques available, rehabilitation has been shown to speed recovery, reduce pain, and prevent contractures. Physiotherapy is important in knee rehabilitation of hemophilic patients and the physiotherapist must work closely with the hematologist (factor coverage) and the orthopedic surgeon.

Arthroscopic synovectomy

At the knee, arthroscopic synovectomy is reserved for the occasion when radiosynovectomy fails to control the synovial membrane (Rodriguez-Merchan 2007b, 2007c; Rodriguez-Merchan *et al.* 2011b).

Arthroscopic synovectomy can be done through at least three portals (anterolateral, anteromedial, and lateral or medial suprapatellar). As complete a synovectomy as possible should be performed with the use of a motorized resector. After arthroscopic synovectomy, the knee should be immobilized in a Robert Jones dressing for 3 days and active movement encouraged. It is a major surgical procedure that requires at least 3 weeks of intense factor coverage.

Advanced hemophilic arthropathy

There are a number of orthopedic procedures that can be carried out in the hemophilic knee when a severe degree of arthropathy is reached (Rodriguez-Merchan 2007b, 2007c; Rodriguez-Merchan *et al.* 2011b). They must all be carried out under adequate factor coverage for around 3 weeks (the time required for complete wound healing).

Curettage of subchondral bone cysts

Some hemophilic patients present with great subchondral cysts on the proximal tibia. When such a cyst is symptomatic and/or of large size,

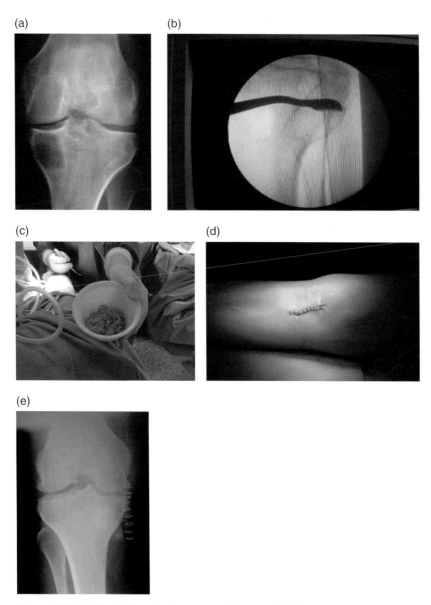

Figure 12.2 Subchondral cyst in the proximal tibia (medial tibial plateau) of a
21-year-old hemophilia patient: (a) Anteroposterior (AP) radiograph showing the cyst.
(b) Intra-operative view: curettage of the cyst with the help of a rongeur under
radioscopy control. (c) Morselized cancellous bone from the Bone Bank ready to fill the
cyst. (d) Surgical incision after closure. (e) Post-operative AP radiograph showing a
satisfactory filling of the cyst.

its curettage and filling with cancellous bone (autologous or from the bone
bank) should be recommended (Rodriguez-Merchan *et al.* 2011b)
(Figure 12.2).

Alignment osteotomies

Sometimes, during childhood, adolescence or early adulthood, some hemophilic knee joints suffer from alteration of their normal axis. Such knees show varus, valgus, or flexion deformities. When the mal-aligned joint is painful and/or severe the patient will need an alignment osteotomy (Rodriguez-Merchan *et al.* 2011b). The most common osteotomies performed in hemophiliacs at the knee are: proximal tibial valgus osteotomy, supracondylar femoral varus osteotomy, and knee extension osteotomy. In all of them, the rationale is to produce a fracture at an adequate area in order to realign the joint to a normal axis. After the osteotomy, it is necessary to adequately fixate the bone using any kind of internal fixation device. Correction of a flexion contracture of the knee has been done at the same time of a spontaneous supracondylar fracture of the femur. When axial malalignment occurs in an adult patient with severe hemophilic arthropathy, a total knee arthroplasty (TKA) would be commonly indicated, and hence both problems can be solved at the same time.

Arthroscopic joint débridement

A joint débridement is commonly performed in patients suffering from severe hemophilic arthropathy whom the orthopaedic surgeon considers to be too young to undergo a TKA. Débridement is a procedure that can alleviate articular pain and bleeding for a number of years, and delays the need of a TKA (Rodriguez-Merchan *et al.* 2011b). An arthroscopic débridement resects the synovial membrane and curettages the articular cartilage of femoral condyles, tibial plateaus, and patella. Some surgeons do not believe in the efficacy of arthroscopic débridement and, therefore, when facing a severe degree of arthropathy in a young patient, they directly proceed to TKA. In many occasions an arthroscopic synovectomy and a débridement are performed together, because hemophilic synovitis and early arthropathy commonly coexist. Again, post-operative rehabilitation is paramount to avoid loss of range of motion (ROM), and should therefore be undertaken along with adequate hematological control in order to avoid rebleedings.

Total knee arthroplasty

Between the second and fourth decades, many hemophilic patients develop severe articular destruction. For the knee, the best solution is a total knee arthroplasty (TKA). The role of a TKA in persons with hemophilia is very important (Rodriguez-Merchan 2007c; Rodriguez-Merchan *et al.* 2011b). Hemophilic patients with uncontrolled human immunodeficiency virus (HIV) are at risk of bacterial and opportunistic infection because of immunosuppression. In these patients, the risk of infection after orthopedic surgery is of considerable concern. Arthroplasty appeared

(a)   (b)

(c)   (d)

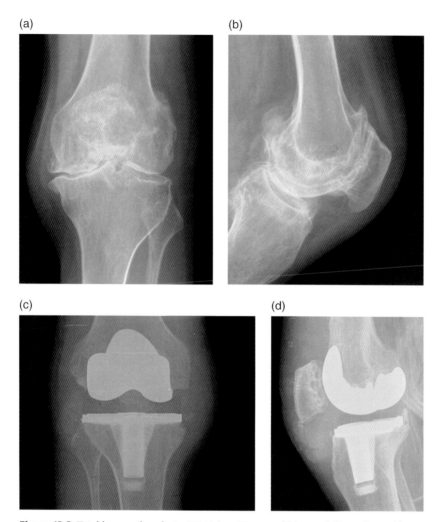

Figure I2.3 Total knee arthroplasty (TKA) in a 42-year-old hemophilia patient with painful severe hemophilic arthropathy: (a) Anteroposterior (AP) pre-operative radiograph. (b) Lateral pre-operative view. (c) AP radiograph 3 years later. (d) Lateral radiograph 3 years later. The short-term result was very satisfactory.

to have seven times the risk of infection as other procedures (Rodriguez-Merchan *et al.* 2011b). TKA for advanced hemophilic arthropathy has good and excellent results in about 85% of cases (Figure I2.3). The main risks are late infection, which can occur regardless of HIV status, and even periprosthetic fracture (Figure I2.4).

Knee flexion contracture

The management of an articular contracture in a patient with hemophilia represents a major challenge. When knee flexion contracture is associated

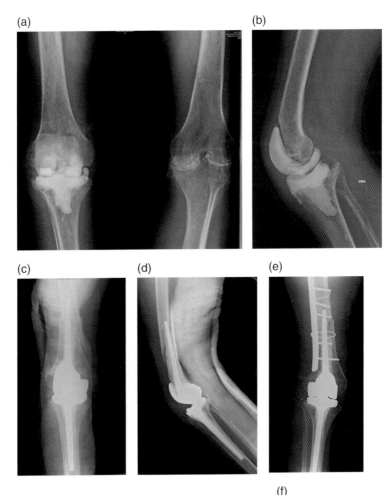

(a)

(b)

(c)

(d)

(e)

Figure 12.4 Infection of TKA in a 48-year-old hemophilia patient that was cured by means of two-stage revision arthroplasty. The case was later complicated by a periprosthetic fracture around the femoral stem. Infection was cured by means of two-stage revision arthroplasty, with an excellent result. However, one year later the patient presented a periprosthetic fracture due to an accidental fall. Then, bone fixation of the periprosthetic fracture was carried out with a satisfactory result: (a) Anteroposterior (AP) radiograph showing the articulated spacer implanted after the removal of the primary TKA (first stage of tw-stage revision arthroplasty for infection). (b) Lateral view of the articulated spacer. (c) AP radiograph showing the revision arthroplasty performed (rotating-hinge prosthesis) in the second stage of revision. Also note a periprosthetic fracture in the distal femur. (d) Lateral radiograph showing the periprosthetic fracture around the femoral stem of the rotating-hinge prosthesis. (e) Good bone fixation was performed by means of plate and screws, supplemented with wires (AP view). (f) Lateral radiograph showing the aforementioned bone fixation.

(f)

with end-stage arthropathy of the knee, a TKA is required (Rodriguez-Merchan *et al.* 2011b). The treatments available for knee flexion contracture are nonoperative (rehabilitation and physiotherapy, orthotics, and corrective devices) and surgical procedures.

Nonoperative treatment

The aim of rehabilitation and physiotherapy is to maintain muscle power and a good ROM. Several specific devices have been used to overcome hemophilic contractures. The most basic of these is the serial application of plaster of paris casts, which are changed approximately weekly as the deformity is gradually overcome. Serial casting can be complicated by skin necrosis, joint cartilage compression, and joint subluxation. More recently, serial casting has been supplemented by the use of reversed dynamic slings and inflatable splints (Flowtron machine, Huntleigh Medical, Luton, England). Reversed dynamic slings require admission to hospital and close supervision, whereas the Flowtron is easy to use and suitable for home treatment. These noninvasive methods are generally successful in only mild contractures, or are used as adjuncts after radical soft-tissue release, to gradually stretch the tight neurovascular structures. Additionally, these methods can cause articular subluxation. An extension/de-subluxation hinge (EDH) device between cylinder casts on a thigh and calf can be used for the treatment of severe knee flexion contractures.

Surgical treatment

Late or severe cases may require surgical correction in the form of soft-tissue procedures, osteotomies or mechanical distraction using external fixators. The soft-tissue procedures (hamstring release at the knee) are often insufficient to gain full correction. In this situation, the chronically contracted vessels and nerves prevent full correction. Regarding osteotomies, supracondylar extension osteotomy of the femur creates a secondary deformity (angulation and shortening) instead of correcting the deformity, and may lead to abnormal joint-loading forces in the ambulatory patient. External fixators can produce gradual joint distraction. These fixators represent a more efficient way to apply forces to the skeletal deformity. Advantages of these techniques include versatility and minimized risk of neurovascular complications. Problems encountered include a rebound phenomenon after the removal of the external fixator, with loss of the temporarily increased total ROM. The results obtained with mechanical distraction external fixators warrant its wider application.

Patients with inhibitors

The development of an inhibitor against factor VIII or factor IX is the most common and most serious complication of factor replacement therapy in

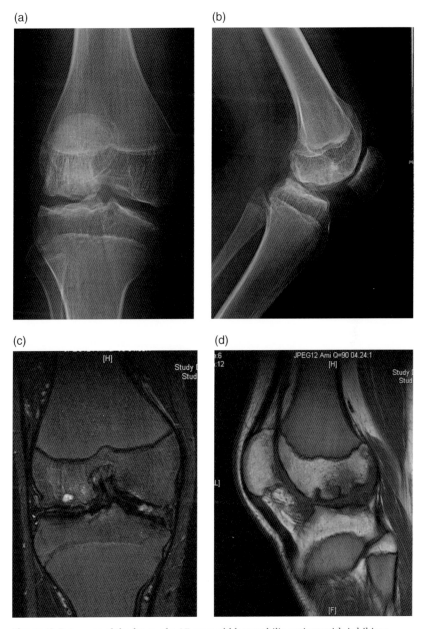

Figure I2.5 Images of the knee of a 17-year-old hemophilia patient with inhibitor, showing a severe degree of hemophilic arthropathy: (a) Anteroposterior (AP) radiograph. (b) Lateral view. (c) MRI of the knee in the AP view. (d) Lateral view of MRI.

patients with hemophilia A or B (Figure I2.5). Recombinant FVIIa and aPCCs have made major elective orthopedic surgery possible in patients with high-titer inhibitors. Previous reports have shown that current

(a)   (b)

(c)   (d)

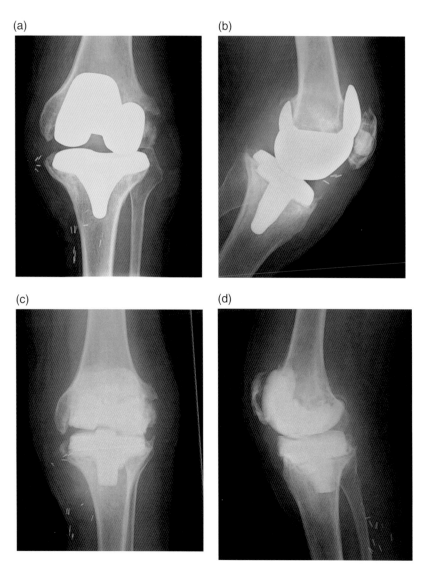

Figure I2.6 Infected TKA in a 54-year-old hemophilia patient with inhibitor:
(a) Anteroposterior (AP) radiograph showing loosening of the components due to
chronic infection of the primary prosthesis. (b) Lateral view showing loosening of the
components. (c) Post-operative view 3 weeks after the removal of the prosthesis and
the implantation of an articulated spacer (first stage of the two-stage revision arthroplasty). (d) Lateral radiograph at 3 weeks showing the articulated spacer. The patient is
waiting for the second stage of revision under intravenous antibiotics treatment.
Normalization of infection parameters (ESR, CRP) is always required before moving on
to the second stage of revision.

hematological advances allows hemophilic patients with inhibitors to undergo surgery with a greater expectation of success, leading to an improved quality of life (Rodriguez-Merchan and Lee 2002; Rodriguez-Merchan *et al.* 2003, 2004, 2007b, 2007c) (Figure I2.6). Thorough analysis of each case as part of a multidisciplinary team will help to identify further inhibitor patients in whom surgery can be performed both safely and effectively. In a publication a consensus was reached regarding the definition of the type of surgical procedures, a scale for evaluating the degree of perioperative bleeding, the recommended doses of FEIBA and rFVIIa for surgery, and the blood tests required before and after surgery (Rodriguez-Merchan *et al.* 2004).

The infectious risk of the HIV-positive patients

HIV-positive hemophilic patients may suffer a spontaneous septic arthritis of the knee that can sometimes mimic a hemarthrosis. The presence of pyrexia and a positive culture of the intra-articular fluid will help us to reach the correct diagnosis. Intravenous antibiotics many times may be sufficient, but it may be necessary to perform surgical drainage and joint lavage of the joint through an arthrotomy. Taking into account that a large proportion of our adult hemophilic population is HIV-positive, their immunological status is likely to be deficient when surgery is considered. Furthermore, most of them also are positive for hepatitis C. In fact, the risk of post-operative infection is higher in hemophilics than in normal patients because of their immunosuppression. However, some controversy exists on this particular point. While some authors have reported a much higher post-operative infection risk in patients with a CD4 count lower than 200/mm^3, others have not found such a high level of infection. Modern treatments against immunodeficiency have made it possible for hemophilic patients to undergo orthopedic surgery with a relatively satisfactory immunological status.

Conclusions

Continuous prophylaxis with factor can halt or slow the development of the orthopedic complications of hemophilia that we still see today. However, this has not been achieved so far, not even in developed countries; therefore, orthopedic surgeons are still needed to carry out many different surgical procedures in the knee. HIV infection has necessitated some immunosuppressed persons to require arthrotomies for the treatment of a spontaneous septic arthritis; moreover, such patients have a high risk of post-operative infection after any surgical procedure, especially a TKA. Current hematological advances allow hemophilic patients with and without inhibitors to undergo knee surgery with a greater expectation of success. Radiosynovectomy is a very effective procedure that decreases both the frequency and the intensity of recurrent intra-articular bleeds related to knee synovitis. The procedure should be performed as soon as possible to minimize the degree of articular cartilage damage. No damage has been reported in relation to the radioactive materials. Personal experience and the general recommendation is that when three early consecutive radiosynovectomies (repeated every 6 months) fail to halt synovitis, an arthroscopic synovectomy should be immediately considered. For advanced hemophilic arthropathy of the knee, the best solution is a TKA. Other surgical (arthroscopic débridement, alignment osteotomy) and non-surgical procedures (rehabilitation, correction devices) are less commonly needed for the hemophilic knee.

References

De la Corte-Rodriguez H, Rodriguez-Merchan EC, Jimenez-Yuste V (2011a) Radiosynovectomy in patients with chronic hemophilic synovitis: when is more than one injection necessary? *Eur J Haematol* **86**: 430–435.

De la Corte-Rodriguez H, Rodriguez-Merchan EC, Jimenez-Yuste V (2011b) Radiosynovectomy in hemophilia: Quantification of its effectiveness through the assessment of 10 articular parameters. *J Thromb Hemost* **9**: 928–935.

De la Corte-Rodriguez H, Rodriguez-Merchan EC, Jimenez-Yuste V (2011c) What patient, joint and isotope characteristics influence the response to radiosynovectomy in patients with hemophilia. *Haemophilia* **17**: e990–998.

Jimenez-Yuste V, Rodriguez-Merchan EC, Alvarez-Roman MT, Martin-Salces M (2011) Prophylaxis in adults with hemophilia. In: Rodriguez-Merchan EC, Valentino LA (eds.), *Current and Future Issues in Hemophilia Care*. Wiley–Blackwell, Oxford, UK, pp. 27–29.

Rodriguez-Merchan EC (2007a) Hemophilic synovitis: basic concepts. *Haemophilia* **13** (Suppl 3): 1–3.

Rodriguez-Merchan EC (2007b) Total joint arthroplasty: the final solution for knee and hip when synovitis could not be controlled. *Haemophilia* **13** (Suppl 3): 49–58.

Rodriguez-Merchan EC (2007c) Total knee replacement in hemophilic arthropathy. *J Bone Joint Surg Br* **89B**: 186–188.

Rodriguez-Merchan EC (2010) Radiosynoviorthesis in hemophilia. In: Lee CA, Berntorp E, Hoots WK (eds.), *Textbook of Hemophilia*. Wiley–Blackwell, Oxford, UK, pp. 182–186.

Rodriguez-Merchan EC, Lee CA (2002) *Inhibitors in Patients with Hemophilia*. Blackwell Science Ltd, Oxford.

Rodriguez-Merchan EC, Wiedel JD, Wallny T, *et al.* (2003) Elective orthopaedic surgery for inhibitors patients. *Haemophilia* **9**: 625–631.

Rodriguez-Merchan EC, Rocino A, Ewenstein B, *et al.* (2004) Consensus perspectives on surgery in hemophilia patients with inhibitors: summary statement. *Haemophilia* **10** (Suppl 2): 50–52.

Rodriguez-Merchan EC, Quintana M, De la Corte-Rodriguez H, Coya M (2007a) Radioactive synoviorthesis for the treatment of hemophilic synovitis. *Hemophilia* **13** (Suppl 3): 32–37.

Rodriguez-Merchan EC, Quintana M, Jimenez-Yuste V, Hernandez-Navarro F (2007b) Orthopaedic surgery for inhibitor patients: a series of 27 procedures (25 patients). *Haemophilia* **13**: 613–619.

Rodriguez-Merchan EC, Valentino L, Quintana M (2007c) Prophylaxis and treatment of chronic synovitis in hemophilia patients with inhibitors. *Haemophilia* 2007c; **13** (Suppl 3): 45–48.

Rodriguez-Merchan EC, Jimenez-Yuste V, Aznar JA, *et al.* (2011a) Joint protection in haemophilia. *Haemophilia* **17**(Suppl 2): 1–23.

Rodriguez-Merchan EC, Jimenez-Yuste V, Goddard NJ (2011b) Initial and advanced stages of hemophilic arthropathy and other musculo-skeletal problems: the role of orthopedic surgery. In: Rodriguez-Merchan EC, Valentino LA (eds.), *Current and Future Issues in Hemophilia Care*. Wiley–Blackwell, Oxford, UK, pp. 127–132.

Valentino LA (2010) Blood-induced joint disease: the pathophysiology of hemophilic arthropathy. *J Thromb Haemost* **8**: 1895–1902.

SECTION II
Hemophilia with Inhibitors

CASE STUDY 1

Inhibitor Patient Requiring High Dose Therapy with rVIIa as well as Sequential Therapy with FEIBA

Alice D. Ma

Division of Hematology/Oncology, University of North Carolina, Chapel Hill, NC, USA

A 30-year-old man from Mexico presented with hematuria. He was wheelchair-bound due to hemiparesis resulting from a traumatic spinal cord bleed at age 3. He had developed a right calf pseudotumor involving the fibular head. He had been treated with cryoprecipitate and red cell transfusions in Mexico until roughly 2003, when factor concentrates became available. He emigrated to the USA in 2006 and presented to the HTC for comprehensive care. He was known to have an FVIII inhibitor which was said to be low titer and low responding. He clinically responded to FVIII infusions.

His initial evaluation at our HTC revealed a Bethesda titer of 5 BU as well as infection with HIV and hepatitis B. He had frequent urinary tract infections due to a neurogenic bladder, requiring intermittent straight catheterization.

The patient underwent a right leg amputation below the knee for control of his expanding pseudotumor with hemostasis provided by FVIII given by continuous infusion. FVIII levels were maintained at 100% for 1 week, then b.i.d. bolus dosing was maintained for a further week. The Bethesda titer rose and peaked at 28 BU. Hemostasis was then maintained using rVIIa.

At the time of this episode, the patient had been dosing with rVIIa, 90–100 mcg/kg every 2 h × 3 doses daily without improvement in hematuria and mild right flank pain. His hemoglobin had fallen from his baseline of 9.5 to 6.6 g/dL. A CT scan of the abdomen and pelvis showed a right ureteral filling defect without other masses or hydronephrosis.

Hemophilia and Hemostasis: A Case-Based Approach to Management, Second Edition.
Edited by Alice D. Ma, Harold R. Roberts, Miguel A. Escobar.
© 2013 John Wiley & Sons, Ltd. Published 2013 by John Wiley & Sons, Ltd.

High doses of rVIIa up to 270 mcg/kg every 2–3 h failed to lead to hemostasis, and he eventually required sequential therapy with APCCs for cessation of hematuria.

Two months later, he was re-admitted due to bilateral deltoid hematomas from immunizations administered in another clinic. He could no longer push himself in his wheelchair, and rVIIa was providing unreliable hemostasis at home. He began ITI with monoclonal FVIII at 100 units/kg b.i.d. He subsequently had no further bleeding episodes, and his Bethesda titer reached 0 within 4 months.

Q1	What are the rationale and the data supporting the use of rVIIa at doses higher than 90–120 mcg/kg?

We presume that the rate of thrombin generation is critical for the formation of a stable fibrin clot. However, the exact relationship between the bolus dose of rVIIa administered and the patient's level of thrombin generation has yet to be defined. Substantial inter-individual variation in thrombin generation has been shown following rVIIa treatment: doses of 90–120 mcg/kg may, in some individuals, be sufficient to produce enough thrombin, whereas other patients may require higher, recurrent dosing.

Dr. Salaj and colleagues (2009) analyzed the bleeding patterns of Czech adult hemophilia patients with high responding inhibitors obtained by the HemoRec registry. In this retrospective analysis, patients who were treated after 2 h of bleeding onset experienced fewer rebleeding episodes when high-dose rVIIa was used (15.8% and 0%; <120 mcg/kg and >250 mcg/kg, respectively). Initial high-dose rVIIa was also associated with a decline in total rVIIa consumption.

A number of case series have also investigated the use of high-dose rVIIa in the treatment of bleeding episodes in inhibitor patients. For example, Kenet and colleagues (2003) assessed the efficacy and safety of a rVIIa "megadose" (300 mcg/kg bolus) as treatment for bleeds in three young inhibitor patients. Of 114 bleeds, 95 responded to a single dose. Pain relief was faster and therapy duration significantly shorter than with continuous infusion (CI) regimens or standard boluses (90 mcg/kg every 3 h). Rebleeding occurred in 9.6% of cases, and 19 of 114 episodes required a second bolus injection. They concluded that treatment of bleeds with a rVIIa megadose in young inhibitor patients is effective and well tolerated.

In summary, some patients clinically fail to respond to standard dose rVIIa. In these patients, it may be reasonable to carefully titrate the dose of rVIIa upward until a clinical response is achieved.

Q2	What are the rationale and the data supporting the use of sequential bypassing agent therapy?

Approximately 10–20% of bleeding episodes cannot be controlled with a single bypassing agent. There have been case reports as well as case series describing the use of rVIIa, followed by an APCC. In these cases, the addition of FXa is felt to contribute to the thrombin generation achieved by rVIIa alone. This has been shown by in vitro experiments on thrombin generation in a cell-based model of hemostasis. This should be considered a salvage maneuver, because of the increased risk of thrombosis. Indeed, elevated D-dimer levels have been seen in some patients treated with this protocol. Drs. Ingerslev and Sørensen (2011) reviewed 17 reports detailing the parallel use of bypassing agents in the same bleeding episode in 49 patients. Five of nine patients with hemophilia developed thrombotic events. Five of 40 patients with congenital hemophilia with inhibitors also had thromboembolic events. Four cases were fatal. If this regimen is used, careful monitoring for thrombotic events is critical.

Q3	When should ITI be considered in an adult inhibitor patient?

In general, immune tolerance therapy (ITI) is most successful when undertaken in patients whose inhibitors have been present for a shorter period of time. Some adult patients have had their inhibitors since childhood, however, without being offered ITI. If these patients experience significant numbers of severe bleeding episodes and have morbidity associated with them, then it is reasonable to consider undertaking ITI. The patient should have no contraindications, such as an inability to adhere to a stringent medical regimen, chronic dental or dermal infections which are likely to lead to CVAD infections, or lack of insurance coverage.

References

Abshire TC (2004) Dose optimization of recombinant factor VIIa for control of mild tomoderate bleeds in inhibitor patients: Improved efficacy with higher dosing. *Semin Hematol* **41**(1 Suppl 1): 3–7. PMID: 1487241.

Gringeri A, Fischer K, Karafoulidou A, *et al.* (2011) European Haemophilia Treatment Standardisation Board (EHTSB). Sequential combined bypassing therapy is safe and effective in the treatment of unresponsive bleeding in adults and children with haemophilia and inhibitors. *Haemophilia* **17**: 630–655. PMID: 21323801.

Ingerslev J, Sørensen B (2011) Parallel use of by-passing agents in haemophilia with inhibitors: a critical review. *Br J Haematol.* Epub ahead of print. PMID: 21895627.

Kenet G, Lubetsky A, Luboshitz J, Martinowitz U (2003) A new approach to treatment of bleeding episodes in young hemophilia patients: a single bolus megadose of recombinant activated factor VII (NovoSeven). *J Thromb Haemos* **1**: 450–455. PMID: 12871449.

Salaj P, Brabec P, Penka M, *et al.* (2009) Effect of rFVIIa dose and time to treatment on patients with haemophilia and inhibitors: analysis of HemoRec registry data from the Czech Republic. *Haemophilia* **15**(3): 752–759. PMID: 19432926.

Schneiderman J, Rubin E, Nugent DJ, Young G (2007) Sequential therapy with activated prothrombin complex concentrates and recombinant FVIIa in patients with severe haemophilia and inhibitors: update of our previous experience. *Haemophilia* **13**: 244–248. PMID: 17498072.

CASE STUDY 2

Prophylactic Therapy in a Patient with a High Titer Inhibitor

Alice D. Ma

Division of Hematology/Oncology, University of North Carolina, Chapel Hill, NC, USA

The patient is a 25-year-old man with mild mental retardation and a history of mild hemophilia A, baseline FVIII level of 6%. In the past, he bled only with trauma and never visited a hemophilia treatment center, receiving all of his care from a community hematologist–oncologist. As a child, he was treated with desmopressin and plasma-derived FVIII. He began having increased traumatic bleeds associated with moving into a group home. These bleeds were treated with recombinant FVIII. More recently, he has been experiencing spontaneous bleeding episodes into his ankles and knees, as well as soft tissue bleeds into his calf and arm muscles. He has been receiving infusions of recombinant FVIII at his doctor's office for his bleeding episodes. His bleeds do not appear to resolve, even with 50 units/kg given daily.

The patient was subsequently referred to the HTC where he was found to have a left ankle bleed. A Bethesda titer was 6 BU.

Over the next 2 months, he had two prolonged (10-day and 13-day) hospital admissions for bleeding episodes that would reccur despite the patient being treated with standard dose rVIIa at 90–100 mcg/kg every 2 h. He eventually required higher dose rVIIa, at 270 mcg/kg, followed in 2 h by 180 mcg/kg q2 h×2.

Q1	How should his inhibitor be eradicated?

Patients with mild/moderate hemophilia A develop inhibitors at lower rates than those with severe hemophilia A, with estimates of inhibitor

---

Hemophilia and Hemostasis: A Case-Based Approach to Management, Second Edition.
Edited by Alice D. Ma, Harold R. Roberts, Miguel A. Escobar.
© 2013 John Wiley & Sons, Ltd. Published 2013 by John Wiley & Sons, Ltd.

development of between 5 and 7%. There are intriguing data, suggesting that these inhibitors may behave more like the autoantibodies seen in acquired hemophilia in terms of their response to immunosuppression. At the University of North Carolina (UNC), our practice has been to treat these patients with Rituximab, 375 mg/m^2 given weekly×4 weeks. We have treated at least 6 individuals with mild/moderate hemophilia A with inhibitors with this regimen, and all patients have responded completely with inhibitor eradication. This patient had complete cessation of spontaneous bleeding and dropped his inhibitor titer to 0 BU within 4 months after completing his course of Rituximab.

Other approaches could include immune tolerance induction, which we have not had to use at UNC for a mild/moderate hemophilia A patient in over a decade.

Q2	Is there any evidence supporting the use of prophylactic treatment with by passing agents?

Dr. Konkle and colleagues (2007) tested rVIIa in secondary prophylaxis of 38 inhibitor patients. These patients received daily rVIIa at either 90 or 270 mcg/kg for 3 months. Bleeding frequency was markedly decreased by 45% and 59%, respectively, which was maintained during the 3-month post-treatment observation period. There was no significant difference between doses.

Dr. Leissinger and colleagues (2011) have recently published the Pro-FEIBA study which was a prospective, randomized crossover study of FEIBA given on demand (OD) or prophylactically (85 U/kg given t.i.w.) for 6 months. Both total bleeds and joint bleeds were significantly reduced during the prophylaxis period compared with the OD period.

References

Franchini M, Salvagno GL, Lippi G (2006) Inhibitors in mild/moderate haemophilia A: an update. *Thromb Haemost* **96**: 113–118.

Konkle BA, Ebbesen LS, Erhardtsen E, *et al.* (2007) Randomized, prospective clinical trial of recombinant factor VIIa for secondary prophylaxis in hemophilia patients with inhibitors. *J Thromb Haemost* **5**: 1904–1913.

Leissinger C, Gringeri A, Antmen B, *et al.* (2011) Anti-inhibitor coagulant complex prophylaxis in hemophilia with inhibitors. *N Engl J Med* **365**(18): 1684–1692.

Peerlinck K, Jacquemin M (2010) Mild haemophilia: a disease with many faces and many unexpected pitfalls. *Haemophilia* **16** (Suppl 5): 100–106.

CASE STUDY 3

Immune Tolerance Induction

Trinh T. Nguyen[1] and Miguel A. Escobar[2]

[1] Division of Hematology, University of Texas Health Science Center at Houston
[2] Gulf States Hemophilia and Thrombophilia Center, Houston, TX, USA

A 9-month-old African American male with severe factor VIII deficiency presented for routine check-up. An inhibitor screen at the time was noted to be 2.55 BU. This was repeated 26 days later and had increased to 5.6 BU.

Of note, he had recently completed 21 days of factor VIII therapy for a spontaneous intracranial hemorrhage and had a port placed during his hospitalization for prolonged factor infusion.

Q1	What are the risk factors of inhibitor development in patients with factor VIII deficiency?

There are genetic, nonmodifiable, risk factors as well as nongenetic, modifiable, risk factors for the development of an inhibitor. Of the risk factors – genetic or not – the single most important factor is the type of gene mutation. Patients with large deletions, nonsense mutations, and inversions are more likely to develop an inhibitor compared to patients with smaller deletions or missense mutations.

The severity of the factor deficiency is also important as most factor VIII deficient patients who develop inhibitors have the severe form of the disease. Ethnicity and family history also add to the risk of inhibitor development. African-Americans, for instance, have a two-fold increased risk compared to Caucasians for inhibitor development. Recent data from the US registry suggests that Hispanics also have a greater risk compared to Caucasians for developing an inhibitor. Having a positive family history of inhibitors increases a patient's risk of inhibitor development more than

Hemophilia and Hemostasis: A Case-Based Approach to Management, Second Edition.
Edited by Alice D. Ma, Harold R. Roberts, Miguel A. Escobar.
© 2013 John Wiley & Sons, Ltd. Published 2013 by John Wiley & Sons, Ltd.

three-fold. Another nongenetic risk factor associated with increased risk of inhibitor development is early exposure to factor – i.e being treated during the first 50 exposure days.

For this patient, risk factors include having a large gene deletion, being of African-American descent, and recently receiving 21 days of therapy for his intracranial bleed. Prior to this, he had only received one dose of factor replacement for a suspected knee bleed.

Other suggested risk factors for inhibitor development include factor replacement during times of stress – known as "danger signals." Certainly for him, the intracranial bleeding and the emergent port placement for IV access were two additional factors that could have increased his risk of inhibitor development.

Approximately 25–33% of severe hemophilia A patients develop inhibitors. In most of these patients, the inhibitor is transient and 5–10% spontaneously resolve. In patients who require therapy, 60–80% respond to immune tolerance induction (ITI).

Q2	What are the prognostic indicators of response to ITI?

Prognostic indicators of response to ITI – the good-risk responders are those with:
- Pre-ITI inhibitor titer <10 BU
- Peak inhibitor titer <200 BU
- <5 years since diagnosis of inhibitor.

Q3	When should immune tolerance induction be initiated?

Typically the decision of when to initiate ITI depends on the patient's BU at the time of diagnosis, as well as the patient's clinical presentation. When possible, it is desirable to avoid further factor VIII exposure and follow the inhibitor titer to <10 BU prior to initiating ITI. Certainly if the patient continues to spontaneously bleed during this waiting period, the decision to initiate ITI may occur at the discretion of the physician and the clinical presentation that necessitates early treatment.

Q4	Which is the best product to use during ITI?

There is no conclusive evidence for the "best" factor VIII product to use for ITI. There are several small-scale studies suggesting that the use of von Willebrand-containing plasma-derived products increases the likelihood of successful ITI compared to recombinant factor VIII products. Meta-analysis of the International Immune Tolerance Study and the North American Immune Tolerance Study, as well as PROFIT study (Italian ITI registry), however, found no association between outcome and treatment product.

Q5	What determines success or failure of ITI?

Successful ITI is defined as:
- undetectable inhibitor level (<0.6 BU/mL)
- factor VIII plasma recovery >66%
- factor VIII half-life >6 h after a 72-h washout
- absence of anamnesis with further factor VIII exposure

and partial success as:
- inhibitor titer <5 BU
- factor VIII recovery <66%
- factor VIII half-life after 72-h washout period of <6 h
- presence of a clinical response to factor VIII
- no increase in the inhibitor titer >5 BU over a 6-month period of on-demand therapy or 12 months of prophylaxis.

Failure of ITI is defined as lack of partial or complete success. This includes
- failure to fulfill criteria for full or partial success within 33 months of therapy
- less than 20% reduction in the inhibitor titer for any 6-month period during ITI after the first 3 months of therapy
- i.e. at least 9 months of ITI have been attempted without reduction of inhibitor titer, and/or
- at most, 33 months ITI attempted.

In practice, however, there are cases of patients who failed to respond to ITI within this 33-month period who were then treated for a longer time and eventually responded. Our patient is a prime example.

References

Astermark J, Lacroix-Desmazes S, Reding MT (2008) Inhibitor development. *Haemophilia* **14**(Suppl 3): 36–42.
Astermark J, Santagostino E, Keith Hoots W (2010) Clinical issues in inhibitors. *Haemophilia* **16**(Suppl 5): 54–60.

DiMichele DM, Hoots WK, Pipe SW, *et al.* (2007) International workshop on immune tolerance induction: consensus recommendations. *Haemophilia* **13**(Suppl 1): 1–22.

Gouw SC, van der Bom JG, Marijke van den Berg H (2007) Treatment-related risk factors of inhibitor development in previously untreated patients with hemophilia A: the Canal cohort study. *Blood* **109**(11): 4648–4654.

Hoyer LW (1995) The incidence of factor VIII inhibitors in patients with severe hemophilia A. *Adv Exp Med Biol* **386**: 35–45.

Miller CH, Platt SJ, Rice AS, *et al.* (2011) F8 and F9 mutations in US haemophilia patients: correlation with history of inhibitor and race/ethnicity. *Haemophilia* Nov 21. doi: 10.1111/j.1365-2516.2011.02700.x. [Epub ahead of print]

Oldenburg J, Brackmann HH, Schwaab R (2000) Risk factors for inhibitor development in hemophilia A. *Haematologica* **85**(Suppl 10): 7–13.

Schwaab R, Brackmann HH, Meyer C, *et al.* (1995) Haemophilia A: mutation type determines risk of inhibitor formation. *J Thromb Haemost* **74**(6): 1402–1406.

CASE STUDY 4

Monitoring During Immune Tolerance Induction

Trinh T. Nguyen[1] and Miguel A. Escobar[2]
[1]Division of Hematology, University of Texas Health Science Center at Houston
[2]Gulf States Hemophilia and Thrombophilia Center, Houston, TX, USA

A 13-month-old Caucasian male with severe factor VIII deficiency presented with pain and swelling of the right ankle. He had received an on-demand dose of factor VIII at home without symptomatic improvement. His mother brought him to the ER where he received another dose of recombinant factor VIII with improvement in symptoms. An inhibitor titer was sent, but as he had responded to the second dose of factor VIII, he was discharged with a follow-up at the HTC in a few days. At follow-up, his Bethesda titer was found to be 9 BU. Immune tolerance induction (ITI) was initiated immediately with follow-up inhibitor titer decreasing to 3 BU in 1 month. However, 3 months into therapy, follow-up inhibitor titer had risen to 38 BU.

Q	How often do you monitor inhibitor titers during ITI?

Clinical indicators of the presence of an inhibitor include a decreased response to factor replacement during therapy for a bleed or bleeding in unusual places. The goal of immune tolerance induction is to allow the body's immune system to become tolerant of the replacement factor VIII and discontinue the formation of antibody inhibitors against the replacement factor.

Once an inhibitor develops, the standard of care is to initiate ITI as soon as possible. For those with inhibitor titers >10 BU, monthly monitoring of the inhibitor titer is warranted until the titer is <10 BU, when ITI commences. Those patients who initiate ITI while the inhibitor titer is still

---

Hemophilia and Hemostasis: A Case-Based Approach to Management, Second Edition.
Edited by Alice D. Ma, Harold R. Roberts, Miguel A. Escobar.
© 2013 John Wiley & Sons, Ltd. Published 2013 by John Wiley & Sons, Ltd.

elevated are less likely to be successfully tolerized. Data from the International Immune Tolerance Study suggests a median of 3 months for inhibitor titers to fall below 10 BU (unpublished).

Once ITI has been initiated, there is no consensus on the frequency of monitoring of inhibitor titers during ITI. It is well known, however, that the inhibitor titer may increase in response to factor VIII re-exposure. This anamnestic response will cause a rise in the Bethesda titer assayed in 3–5 days. As such, at our center, we typically monitor the inhibitor titer within a month of therapy and continue monthly titers until there is a steady downward trend. We then decrease the frequency of monitoring to every 3 months until (successful) completion of therapy.

Reference

Hay CR, *et al.* (2006) The diagnosis and management of factor VIII and IX inhibitors: a guideline from the United Kingdom Haemophilia Centre Doctors Organisation. *Br J Haematol* **133**(6): 591–605.

CASE STUDY 5

Factor IX Inhibitors

Trinh T. Nguyen[1] and Miguel A. Escobar[2]
[1]Division of Hematology, University of Texas Health Science Center at Houston
[2]Gulf States Hemophilia and Thrombophilia Center, Houston, TX, USA

An 11-year-old Filipino boy with severe factor IX deficiency developed a high titer inhibitor during therapy for a traumatic subdural hematoma at 3 years of age. He received recombinant factor VIIa during his hospitalization which continued × 21 days total. This was changed to daily prophylactic dosing ~100–150 mcg/kg/dose. Peak inhibitor titer was 72 BU during the acute phase of intracranial bleeding, but slowly trended down. Factor IX was held while waiting for the inhibitor titer to fall below 10 BU prior to initiating ITI. At a nadir, the inhibitor titer was 2.55 BU. Five months later it was decided to start a modified low-dose ITI regimen with recombinant factor IX, 50 units/kg/dose t.i.w. He responded rapidly to immune therapy with negative titers by 3 months of therapy. Unfortunately, due to poor adherence, the inhibitor titer trended up at follow-up 8 months after ITI was initiated.

Clinically, he had occasional traumatic bleeds that responded well to recombinant factor VIIa as needed. Notably, he did not have increased bleeding as his inhibitor titers rose. Hence, ITI was continued in an attempt to eradicate the inhibitor.

Unfortunately, the titer was never <10 BU again, and in fact continued to rise during ITI, peaking at 63.6 BU. After >36 months of therapy, given the persistence of the high-titer inhibitor, ITI was discontinued.

Unfortunately for this patient with a high-titer inhibitor, his disease course has been complicated by recurrent traumatic-intracranial hemorrhages – a total of 4: 2 pre- and 2 post-ITI attempts. Daily prophylaxis with recombinant factor VIIa was continued, but after a third intracranial hemorrhage, which appeared spontaneous in nature, he was switched to thrice weekly dosing with FEIBA prophylaxis 75 units/kg/dose.

Hemophilia and Hemostasis: A Case-Based Approach to Management, Second Edition.
Edited by Alice D. Ma, Harold R. Roberts, Miguel A. Escobar.
© 2013 John Wiley & Sons, Ltd. Published 2013 by John Wiley & Sons, Ltd.

Q1	What is the frequency of inhibitor development in factor IX deficient patients?

Factor IX deficient patients have a much lower risk of inhibitor development compared to factor VIII deficient patients; 10–15% of all factor VIII deficient patients compared to 1–3% of factor IX deficient patients develop inhibitors. Due to the rarity of inhibitor development in factor IX deficient patients, as well as the smaller number of patients with this disease in general, there are few large-scale studies available to appropriately guide preventive and therapeutic strategies for factor IX inhibitor treatment. Much of what is practiced is extrapolated from factor VIII deficient patients. As such, ITI remains the definitive therapy of choice; however, as above, there is no established dosing regimen for factor IX inhibitor eradication.

Q2	What is the treatment of choice for patients with inhibitors to factor IX?

For those select few who develop factor IX inhibitors, the response rate to ITI is poor compared to factor VIII patients who develop inhibitors. In addition, 50% of patients with factor IX inhibitors develop severe allergic reactions, anaphylactoid reactions, and/or frank anaphylaxis. In addition, patients who have allergic reactions are also at risk of developing potentially irreversible nephrotic syndrome. The risk is such that some institutions actually admit the patients and monitor them for anaphylaxis with the first several doses of factor IX during ITI.

Reference

DiMichele DM (2011) Immune tolerance induction in haemophilia: evidence and the way forward. *J Thromb Haemost* **9**(Suppl 1): 216–225.

CASE STUDY 6

Severe Hemophilia B with High Response Inhibitor and Anaphylactic Reaction to Factor IX

Jenny M. Splawn,[1] *Benjamin Carcamo,*[2] *and Miguel A. Escobar*[3]

[1]Providence Memorial Hospital, El Paso, TX, USA

[2]Pediatric Hematology Oncology, Providence Memorial Hospital, and Texas Tech University School of Medicine, El Paso, TX, USA

[3]Division of Hematology, University of Texas Health Science Center at Houston and Gulf States Hemophilia and Thrombophilia Center, Houston, TX, USA

The patient was diagnosed at 6 months of age with severe factor IX deficiency after presenting with several large subcutaneous, soft tissue, and intramuscular hematomas. He began treatment on demand with recombinant factor IX. Following a port a-cath placement at 2 years of age, he developed a large subcutaneous chest hematoma which failed to respond to high-dose recombinant factor IX. He was subsequently found to have high-titer factor IX inhibitor (12.0 BU) and was treated with recombinant factor VIIa (rFVII) to manage his symptoms.

Immune tolerance induction (ITI) with recombinant factor IX (FIX) was attempted at age 4. However, the patient developed flushing, tightening of the throat, and a strong anamnestic response (FIX inhibitor of 77 BU). FIX therapy was discontinued. One month later, he received a dose of an aPCC, FEIBA, and developed fever and chest pain.

With apparent rejection of FIX and bypass therapy with FEIBA, the patient continued receiving rFVIIa for the management of his bleeding episodes. His bleeds did not respond adequately to the standard doses of 90–20 mcg/kg, requiring doses of up to 420 mcg/kg IV every 6–12 h as prophylaxis, and an additional 630 mcg/kg IV every 2 h for acute bleeding. His school absenteeism had increased with a decline in quality of life due to frequent bleeding episodes and hospitalizations, despite high doses of rFVIIa.

Hemophilia and Hemostasis: A Case-Based Approach to Management, Second Edition. Edited by Alice D. Ma, Harold R. Roberts, Miguel A. Escobar.
© 2013 John Wiley & Sons, Ltd. Published 2013 by John Wiley & Sons, Ltd.

Q	How should this patient be managed next?

At the age of 9 it was decided to attempt desensitization with the use of rituximab and steroids. Informed consent was obtained from the patient and his parents. The patient was admitted to the pediatric intensive care unit under anaphylactic precautions. Baseline aPTT was 102 s. He received rituximab at 375 mg/m^2, and was continuously monitored throughout the infusion. He began the FIX desensitization protocol modified from Dioun *et al.* (1998) and Chuansumrit *et al.* (2008) (Table 6.1). The cumulative dose for each day was 100 units/kg of recombinant FIX.

Table 6.1 Desensitization protocol.

Dose (units/kg)			
Pre-ITI	FIX	Method	Concentration
Day 1	0.01	Slow IV push	0.25 units
	0.02	Slow IV push	0.5 units
	0.04	Slow IV push	1 unit
	0.08	Slow IV push	2 units
	0.1	Slow IV push	2.5 units
	0.2	Slow IV push	5 units
	0.4	Slow IV push	10 units
	0.8	Slow IV push	20 units
	1.5	Slow IV push	37 units
	3	IV over 30 min	75 units
	6	IV over 30 min	150 units
	8	IV over 30 min	200 units
	9	IV over 60 min	222 units
	11	IV over 60 min	275 units
	12	IV over 60 min	300 units
	14	IV over 60 min	350 units
	16	IV over 60 min	400 units
	18	IV over 60 min	450 units
Day 2	100	IV over 10 h	2470 units
Day 3	100	IV over 8 h	2470 units

Table 6.1 (*cont'd*)

Dose (units/kg)			
Pre-ITI	FIX	Method	Concentration
Day 4	100	IV over 6 h	2470 units
Day 5	100	IV over 4 h	2470 units
Day 6	100	IV over 2 hours	2470 units
Day 7	100	IV over 1 h	2470 units
Day 8	100	IV over 30 min	2470 units

Table 6.2 Coagulation studies before and after ITI.

	FIX Inhibitor	aPTT	FIX activity	FIX dose
Pre-ITT	<0.8 BU	102	<0.5	–
Day 4	–	36.3	–	100 units/kg/day
Day 300	<0.8 BU	59	26.4	100 units/kg/day

On the first day of desensitization, the patient experienced a rash with urticaria near the infusion site. The symptoms resolved quickly after administration of diphenhydramine and hydrocortisone. The subsequent days of infusion were well tolerated. Following Day 8 of infusion, the patient was given a 1 gm/kg dose of intravenous immune globulin, and was started on mycophenolate mofetil at 600 mg/m² twice daily for 1 month. The patient received a further three doses of once weekly rituximab, and continued to receive 100 units/kg of recombinant FIX daily.

Eleven months after ITI, the patient was hospitalized for an acute febrile illness. After 10 days of antibiotic therapy, the patient returned home. He has required no further hospitalizations for either an opportunistic infection or management of bleeds. Over a year after completion of immune tolerance therapy with rituximab, this patient has continued to receive recombinant factor IX without allergic reaction or nephrotic syndrome. His inhibitor titer remains negative and he continues to receive prophylaxis with recombinant FIX once a day (Table 6.2).

Patients with severe hemophilia B and inhibitors are rare. Thus, there are few case reports of successful ITI in these patients. A subset of these patients develop allergic reactions to FIX that further complicates treatment. They usually are unable to tolerate PCC and aPCCs since these products contain significant amounts of FIX. The best means of eradication of the antibody is through ITI. ITI uses daily infusion of the deficient factor (FIX) until the inhibitor is no longer present. The addition of rituximab, an anti-CD20 monoclonal antibody, to ITI has been shown to be effective in patients with hemophilia B and inhibitors. Potential complications have been associated with ITI, including anaphylactic reactions and nephrotic syndrome.

References

Alexander S, Hopewell S, Hunter S, *et al.* (2008) Rituximab and desensitization for a patient with severe factor IX deficiency, inhibitors, and history of anaphylaxis. *J Pediatr Hematol Oncol* **30**: 93–95.

Chuansumrit A, Moonsup Y, Sirachainan N, *et al.* (2008) The use of rituximab as an adjuvant for immune tolerance therapy in a hemophilia B boy with inhibitor and anaphylaxis to factor IX concentrate. *Blood Coagul Fibrinolysis* **19**: 208–211.

Dioun AF, Ewenstein BM, Geha RS, Schneider LC (1998) IgE-mediated allergy and desentization to factor IX in hemophilia B. *J Allergy Clin Immunol* **102**: 113–117.

Shibata M, Shima M, Misu H, *et al.* (2003) Management of haemophilia B inhibitor patients with anaphylactic reactions to FIX concentrates. *Haemophilia* **9**: 269–271.

Tengborn L, Hansson S, Fasth A, *et al.* (1998) Anaphylactoid reactions and nephritic syndrome – a considerable risk during factor IX treatment in patients with hemophilia B and inhibitors: a report on the outcome in two brothers. *Haemophilia* **4**: 854–859.

Warrier I, Ewenstein BM, Koerper MA, *et al.* (1997) Factor IX inhibitors and anaphylaxis in hemophilia B. *J Pediatr Hematol Oncol* **19**: 23–27.

CASE STUDY 7

Inhibitor Patient and Dental Surgery

Alice D. Ma

Division of Hematology/Oncology, University of North Carolina, Chapel Hill, NC, USA

A 50-year-old African-American man with severe hemophilia A and a history of a high-responding, high-titer inhibitor presented with severe dental caries and the need for a full mouth extraction. He was known to respond well to rVIIa at standard doses of 90–120 mcg/kg. Pre-operatively, the patient was treated with epsilon aminocaproic acid, 50 mg/kg IV, as well as rVIIa at 120 mcg/kg. The epsilon aminocaproic acid was continued every 6 h and the rVIIa was given every 2 h until 24 h after the procedure, then was decreased to every 4 h. Despite these measures, hemostasis was poor. The patient became hypotensive to a BP of 75/53. A large mandibular hematoma formed and caused swelling of his lips and neck, without airway compromise (see Figure 7.1). Two units of PRBC were transfused. Hemostasis was eventually achieved by day 7, and the patient was discharged by the covering hematologist. However, at home, the patient had persistent bleeding, and required re-admission. On his way back to the hospital, his car was rear-ended by a pickup truck, and the patient suffered open, comminuted fractures of both femurs. He underwent emergent surgical repair of his femurs under coverage with rVIIa.

Q	What is the optimal therapy for an inhibitor patient who needs to have dental surgery?

Unlike hemophilics without inhibitors who may need only a single dose of FVIII or FIX pre-operatively, along with an antifibrinolytic such as epsilon-aminocaproic acid (amicar) or tranexamic acid, the experience at

---

Hemophilia and Hemostasis: A Case-Based Approach to Management, Second Edition.
Edited by Alice D. Ma, Harold R. Roberts, Miguel A. Escobar.
© 2013 John Wiley & Sons, Ltd. Published 2013 by John Wiley & Sons, Ltd.

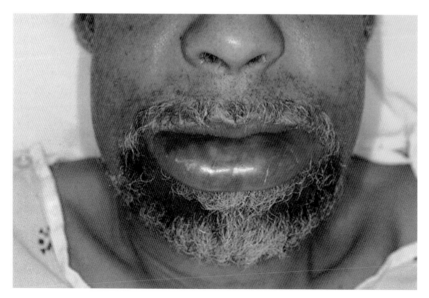

Figure 7.1 Notice the swelling of the lips and neck from pooled blood 24 h after the procedure.

our center suggests that inhibitor patients have significantly more hemorrhagic complications. Even the patients who typically have excellent responses to bypassing agents have more hemorrhage than expected at the time of the procedure, as well as significant delayed post-operative bleeding. We suggest that a bypassing agent be used for 5–7 days (rFVIIa 100 mcg/kg q2 h or FEIBA 100 units/kg q6–8h) along with an antifibrinolytic agent until optimal hemostasis is achieved. Antifibrinolytics should be continued for a total of 10–14 days. At the first sign of rebleeding, bypassing agents should immediately be restarted.

SECTION III
Hemophilic Treatment for Procedures

CASE STUDY 8

Deep Vein Thrombosis Prophylaxis in Patients with Hemophilia A Undergoing Orthopedic Surgery

Alice D. Ma

Division of Hematology/Oncology, University of North Carolina, Chapel Hill, NC, USA

A 60-year-old man with severe hemophilia A presented for elective right total knee arthroplasty. There was no history of inhibitor. He had type 2 diabetes mellitus and hypertension.

Q	How should he be prophylaxed against venous thromboembolism?

Prophylaxis against venous thromboembolism (VTE) in the hemophilic population is a contentious topic. It had been assumed that hemophilics undergoing orthopedic surgery did not require prophylaxis against VTE because of their low risk of thromboembolic disease. Recent data has suggested that while symptomatic VTE is rare, hemophilics undergoing orthopedic surgery have a 10% rate of subclinical VTE.

A survey of practices in hemophilia treatment centers was recently published. Pradhan and colleagues (2009) sent a four-question survey to 140 federally funded hemophilia treatment centers about their practice of VTE prophylaxis. Sixty centers replied. The first question asked if they believed that patients with hemophilia who undergo hip/knee arthroplasty, and are on factor replacement therapy, are at high enough risk for deep vein thrombosis to warrant some type of thromboprophylaxis: 67% responded affirmatively; 25% responded negatively; and 8% responded that this question was not applicable, given that they predominantly managed pediatric patients who rarely undergo joint replacement. Question 2 asked

Hemophilia and Hemostasis: A Case-Based Approach to Management, Second Edition.
Edited by Alice D. Ma, Harold R. Roberts, Miguel A. Escobar.
© 2013 John Wiley & Sons, Ltd. Published 2013 by John Wiley & Sons, Ltd.

if the respondant provided thromboprophylaxis to all hemophilia patients on factor replacement therapy undergoing hip or knee arthroplasty. Of the 67% in support of prophylaxis, 55% answered "yes" and 45% responded "no." Thus, among Hemophilia Treatment Centers, there clearly exists a clinical equipoise with respect to the use of thromboprophylaxis in this setting. The third question asked, of those who did not prophylax all patients, if they provided thromboprophylaxis to selected hemophilia patients on factor replacement therapy undergoing hip or knee arthroplasty (e.g. only if their respective FVIII or FIX levels are above a certain cut-off point, e.g. >100% activity?). Of the 45% of providers who do not provide thromboprophylaxis to all patients, 78% provide prophylaxis to selected patients only if clotting factor levels were above a certain point and 22% provided no thromboprophylaxis. The final question addressed the modality of thromboprophylaxis used. Of those providing thromboprophylaxis, 32% reported using compression stockings, 35% were using sequential compression devices, and 24% reported using low molecular weight heparin, 1% fondaparinux, 3% unfractionated heparin, 4% warfarin, and 1% aspirin.

The practice in our center is to keep the factor VIII or IX concentration between 80 and 100% for the first 5–7 days using continuous infusion. During this time frame, we use low molecular weight heparin for prophylaxis in most patients. Those individuals at high risk for bleeding (e.g. inhibitor patients) receive only prophylaxis with sequential pneumatic compression devices.

References

Hermans C, Hammer F, Lobet S, Lambert C (2010) Subclinical deep venous thrombosis observed in 10% of hemophilic patients undergoing major orthopedic surgery. *J Thromb Haemost* **8**: 1138–1140.

Pradhan SM, Key NS, Boggio L, Pruthi R (2009) Venous thrombosis prophylaxis in haemophilics undergoing major orthopaedic surgery: a survey of haemophilia treatment centres. *Haemophilia* **15**: 1337–1338.

Prostate Surgery and Hemophilia

Alice D. Ma

Division of Hematology/Oncology, University of North Carolina, Chapel Hill, NC, USA

A 68-year-old man with severe hemophilia A presented with urinary symptoms and was recommended to undergo transurethral resection of the prostate (TURP). He has a history of hepatitis C which was successfully eradicated 7 years ago. He has hypertension and gout.

Q	How should the patient be managed from a hemophilia standpoint around the time of his procedure?

Surgery involving the prostate and urinary system is more hemorrhagic due to the presence of urokinase in the invaded tissues. For this reason, the recommendations are to keep the factor VIII levels higher than for other nonurinary surgical procedures. We recommend the use of a FVIII bolus of 50 units/kg, followed by the use of a continuous infusion at 4 units/kg/h. We recommend that the FVIII level be checked 30–60 minutes after the bolus and that it be between 90 and 100% before proceeding to surgery. We recommend that the continuous infusion be maintained for 7–10 days post-operatively. The rate of continuous infusion should be adjusted, based on once or twice daily FVIII activity levels.

Hemophilia and Hemostasis: A Case-Based Approach to Management, Second Edition.
Edited by Alice D. Ma, Harold R. Roberts, Miguel A. Escobar.
© 2013 John Wiley & Sons, Ltd. Published 2013 by John Wiley & Sons, Ltd.

Mild Hemophilia and Intraocular Injections

Alice D. Ma

Division of Hematology/Oncology, University of North Carolina, Chapel Hill, NC, USA

A 68-year-old man with mild hemophilia A, baseline FVIII level of 12%, and documented coronary artery disease, on aspirin presented with intraocular hemorrhage. He had been receiving weekly intraocular injections of bevacizumab without factor replacement prior to the injections. Neither the patient nor his ophthalmologist had informed the HTC about the injections.

Q	How should the patient's intraocular injections be managed in the future?

VEGF inhibitors such as bevacizumab are being given intraocularly for a variety of ophthalmologic conditions, including diabetic retinopathy, macular degeneration, pterygium, among others. However efficacious these agents may be, they have a variety of complications, some of which are thrombotic and others hemorrhagic. This patient has a congenital hemorrhagic disorder and is also on an antiplatelet agent. Though bevacizumab has been given safely in patients who are systemically anticoagulated, some patients have suffered severe hemorrhage. For this reason, we would recommend that the patient receive FVIII injections sufficient to bring the FVIII activity level to above 50% prior to the intraocular injections.

References

Brouzas D, Koutsandrea C, Moschos M, *et al.* (2009) Massive choroidal hemorrhage after intravitreal administration of bevacizumab (Avastin) for AMD followed by controlateral sympathetic ophthalmia. *Clin Ophthalmol* **3**: 457–459.

Hemophilia and Hemostasis: A Case-Based Approach to Management, Second Edition.
Edited by Alice D. Ma, Harold R. Roberts, Miguel A. Escobar.
© 2013 John Wiley & Sons, Ltd. Published 2013 by John Wiley & Sons, Ltd.

Krishnan R, Goverdhan S, Lochhead J (2009) Submacular haemorrhage after intravitreal bevacizumab compared with intravitreal ranibizumab in large occult choroidal neovascularization. *Clin Experi Ophthalmol* **37**(4): 384–388.

Lambert C, Deneys V, Pothen D, Hermans C (2008) Safety of bevacizumab in mild haemophilia B. *Thromb Haemost* **99**(5): 963–964.

Mason JO 3rd, Frederick PA, Neimkin MG, *et al.* (2010) Incidence of hemorrhagic complications after intravitreal bevacizumab (avastin) or ranibizumab (lucentis) injections on systemically anticoagulated patients. *Retina* **30**(9): 1386–1389.

CASE STUDY 11

Endoscopy/Colonoscopy and Hemophilia

Alice D. Ma

Division of Hematology/Oncology, University of North Carolina, Chapel Hill, NC, USA

A 51-year-old man with mild hemophilia A, baseline factor level of 7% is scheduled for routine screening colonoscopy. He does not treat himself with factor at home, and his response to DDAVP shows that his FVIII level rises to 15% at 1 h after desmopressin.

Q	What is the recommendation for factor replacement around the time of his procedure?

Given that this patient does not treat himself at home, we are more conservative, and would opt to treat this gentleman to 80–100% FVIII prior to the procedure. This should be sufficient if no invasive procedures are done during the colonoscopy.

If any biopsies are performed or polyps removed, we would recommend that he be treated to 80–100% on post-procedure days 1 and 3. We would also recommend that he take epsilon aminocaproic acid, 50 mg/kg every 6 h for 7–10 days after the procedure.

Hemophilia and Hemostasis: A Case-Based Approach to Management, Second Edition.
Edited by Alice D. Ma, Harold R. Roberts, Miguel A. Escobar.
© 2013 John Wiley & Sons, Ltd. Published 2013 by John Wiley & Sons, Ltd.

CASE STUDY 12

Dialysis and Hemophilia

Alice D. Ma

Division of Hematology/Oncology, University of North Carolina, Chapel Hill, NC, USA

A 47-year-old man with moderate hemophilia A, severe hemophilic arthropathy, chronic hepatitis C, sleep apnea, gout, and hypertension has developed worsening renal insufficiency with an estimated GFR of 17 mL/min. He had a ruptured viscus at age 25 as a complication of cocaine use. He is on prophylaxis with recombinant FVIII at 30 units/kg t.i.w.

Q1	What is the optimal renal replacement therapy for this gentleman?

Renal disease is quite prevalent in patients with hemophilia. In a meta-analysis of 3,422 hemophilia records, 2,975 persons with hemophilia were documented to have chronic renal disease (52%) or acute renal disease (48%). HIV infection, hypertension, diabetes, and older age were associated with increased renal disease in this population. Hepatitis C infection also doubles the risk of developing renal disease.

   The optimal renal replacement therapy must be individualized for each patient. There are a number of pros and cons to each form of therapy. Peritoneal dialysis can be done at home and offers more stable renal replacement, with exchanges being done 4 times daily, 7 days per week. This form of therapy has been recommended for most hemophilics since it does not require heparinization. However, patients with severe liver disease are not optimal candidates for this mode of dialysis since ascites may interfere with the filtration. Patients with other immunodeficiencies may be at higher risk of infection. This patient, with a history

---

Hemophilia and Hemostasis: A Case-Based Approach to Management, Second Edition.
Edited by Alice D. Ma, Harold R. Roberts, Miguel A. Escobar.
© 2013 John Wiley & Sons, Ltd. Published 2013 by John Wiley & Sons, Ltd.

of a ruptured viscus, may have adhesions limiting the space available for intraperitoneal dialysis.

Hemodialysis done thrice weekly at an outpatient dialysis center is more problematic for most hemophilic patients, due, in large part, to the use of heparin. The optimal use of clotting factor (before, after, during) around the time of dialysis treatment has not been determined. The constant accessing and de-accessing of AV fistulas is a hemostatic challenge, and the administration of a clotting factor through a venous access device or AV fistula is a thrombotic risk. Though hemodialysis can be performed at home, its use has not been reported in a hemophilic population.

Q2	How should we treat him with factor replacement around the time of his dialysis access placement?

Peritoneal dialysis – Rao (2001) recommended replacing clotting factor to 100% for placement of the peritoneal catheter but did not recommend factor replacement during subsequent dialysis treatments. Kothapalli (1989) reported the case of a 27-year-old man with severe hemophilia A in whom factor VIII was given pre-operatively and for 1 week post-operatively for peritoneal catheter placement for 1 week, without bleeding episodes. Peritoneal dialysis was successful without concomitant factor replacement except on two occasions where blood-tinged peritoneal fluid was identified. Factor dose recommendations were not addressed. We favor this latter approach. Additionally, since patients may be uremic, desmopressin may be required pre-operatively to correct uremic platelet dysfunction.

Hemodialysis – Roy-Chaudhury *et al.* (1993) reported 4 of 7 hemophilia cases dialyzed through an arteriovenous (AV) shunt rather than an AV fistula. At that time, there was concern about potential hemorrhage and hematoma formation with repeated access of an AV fistula in hemophilia patients. Factor correction to 100% during the intra-operative phase for vascular access, followed by 50% for the following 5 days was recommended with no bleeding episodes encountered .

Most centers use a combination of heparin during dialysis, as well as FVIII given before and after dialysis. A typical regimen identified is 1,000 units of factor before and after dialysis, with heparin administered continuously in the arterial end of the extracorporeal circulation. Protamine is infused into the venous end to neutralize the heparin effect before blood is returned to the patient.

References

Kothapalli SR (1989) Peritoneal dialysis in a patient with heamophilia and chronic renal failure. *Postgrad Med J* **64**: 506.

Kulkarni R, Soucie J, Evatt B (2003) Renal disease among males with hemophilia. *Haemophilia* **9**: 703–710.

Lambing A, Kuriakose P, Lanzon J, Kachalsky E (2009) Dialysis in the haemophilia patient: a practical approach to care. *Haemophilia* **15**: 33–42.

Rao TKS (2001) Human immunodeficiency virus infection and renal failure. *Infec Dis Clin North Am* **15**: 833–850.

Roy-Chaudhury P, Propper DJ, Catto GRD (1993) Renal replacement therapy for hemophiliacs. *J Nephrol* **6**: 93–94.

CASE STUDY 13

Circumcision

Nidra Rodriguez

Division of Hematology, The University of Texas Health Science Center at Houston and Gulf States
Hemophilia & Thrombophilia Center, MD Anderson Cancer Center, Houston, TX, USA

Q	A newborn male has severe hemophilia A. Can he be circumcised safely?

Circumcision is likely the oldest procedure known and possibly the only surgical procedure performed at parental request. It is primarily performed for religious, social, or cultural reasons and less commonly due to medical reasons. The incidence of post-operative bleeding in hemophilic patients undergoing any type of surgical procedure is approximately 15–20%. Even in males without hemophilia, the most common complication of circumcision is bleeding, with an incidence of 0.1–35%. There are a limited number of publications regarding bleeding post-circumcision in patients with hemophilia. The bleeding risk in such limited cases ranges between 23 and 52%. The risk can be increased by other factors such as severity of hemophilia, presence of an inhibitor, type/extent of surgery, presence of another bleeding disorder, history of prior post-operative hemorrhage, etc. Therefore, it is important to individualize care and take adequate precautions prior to circumcision. Treatment options used to prevent bleeding include factor VIII or IX replacement pre- and post- operatively, antifibrinolytic agents, desmopressin, and fibrin glue among the most commonly described. Even though patients with hemophilia have an increased risk of post-operative bleeding, circumcision can be performed safely as long as adequate measures are in place and factor replacement is administered pre- and post-operatively.

It is important to counsel parents that most insurance companies do not cover routine circumcision without a medical indication, which is felt to be a "cosmetic" procedure.

Hemophilia and Hemostasis: A Case-Based Approach to Management, Second Edition.
Edited by Alice D. Ma, Harold R. Roberts, Miguel A. Escobar.
© 2013 John Wiley & Sons, Ltd. Published 2013 by John Wiley & Sons, Ltd.

References

Kavakli K, Aledort LM (1998) Circumcision and haemophilia: a perspective. *Haemophilia* **4**: 1–3.

Rodriguez V, Titapiwatanakun R, Moir C, *et al.* (2010) To circumcise or not to circumcise? Circumcision in patients with bleeding disorders. *Haemophilia* **16**: 272–276.

Sasmaz I, Antmen B, Leblebisatan G, *et al.* Circumcision and complications in patients with haemophilia in southern part of Turkey: Cukurova experience. *Haemophilia* Dec 2011 (Epub ahead of print).

Shittu OB, Shokunbi WA (2001) Circumcision in haemophiliacs: the Nigerian experience. Haemophilia **7**: 534–536.

Zulfikar B, Ihsan Karaman M, Ovali F (2005) Circumcision in hemophilia: an overview. *Guidelines for the Management of Haemophilia*. World Federation of Hemophilia.

CASE STUDY 14

Pharmacokinetic Studies for Surgery

Miguel A. Escobar

Associate Professor of Medicine and Pediatrics, Division of Hematology, University of Texas Health Science Center at Houston; Director, Gulf States Hemophilia and Thrombophilia Center, Houston, TX, USA

A 57-year-old Caucasian male with severe hemophilia A without inhibitor, and chronic arthropathy, was scheduled for a right total knee replacement. He also had a history of chronic hepatitis C without evidence of cirrhosis. He had been cleared by hepatology and anesthesia to undergo the procedure.

Q	What are the different options to treat this patient and how can the dose of factor required be calculated?

For patients who must undergo elective major surgical procedures, a recovery and half-life study is recommended and should be performed during a non-bleeding state with a 3–5 half-life washout period. A dose of the therapeutic product is infused to increase the plasma level to 100% and samples for factor activity should be drawn at different time intervals: 0, 30, 60 min; 3, 6, 9, 24, and 48 h post-infusion. For FIX additional time points to include 50 and 72 h should be drawn, given the longer half-life. Less number of samples can be obtained when using population PK and Bayesian computer programs to calculate adequate dosing.

Based on the individual's pharmacokinetic study, an initial "loading" dose and subsequent doses can be calculated. For example, in an individual with factor VIII deficiency and a normal recovery and half-life, the dose of factor can be calculated using the following formula:

$$\text{Initial loading dose} = (\text{Desired factor VIII level} - \text{Patient baseline factor VIII})$$
$$\times \text{Body weight}(\text{kg}) \times 0.5 \,\text{unit/kg}.$$

Hemophilia and Hemostasis: A Case-Based Approach to Management, Second Edition.
Edited by Alice D. Ma, Harold R. Roberts, Miguel A. Escobar.
© 2013 John Wiley & Sons, Ltd. Published 2013 by John Wiley & Sons, Ltd.

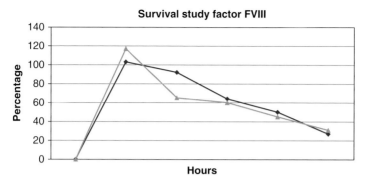

Figure 14.1 Example of two different pharmacokinetic studies with recombinant factor VIII.

Assuming that, 8–12 h after the initial bolus, the plasma level will decrease by about 50%, further doses can be given by one-half of the loading dose every 8–12 h. If a continuous infusion is employed, the initial loading dose should be divided by 12 (half-life of factor VIII), which is equal to the number of units per hour of factor VIII concentrate. For example, to raise the factor VIII level to 100% in a 80-kg individual with less than 1% activity, the initial loading dose will be 4,000 units followed by boluses of 2,000 units every 8–12 h. If a continuous infusion is used, 333 units per hour will be the calculated dose. Factor VIII levels should be monitored daily and ongoing dosing adjusted accordingly.

The dose calculations for factor IX concentrates are different from those used in factor VIII deficiency because the recovery of infused factor IX is lower (~50%) due to the diffusion over a larger volume. To raise to 100% of normal in a 80-kg severely affected patient, 8,000 units should be given as a bolus, followed by half of this amount every 12 to 18 h. The continuous infusion dosing can be calculated by dividing the loading dose by 18–24, i.e. approximately 333 units of factor IX per hour.

For those patients with a rapid initial phase decay or consumption (more than 50% decline in 6 h), a second bolus can be given of factor VIII or factor IX respectively (approximately 50% of initial bolus) within 3–6 h of starting the surgery to avoid excessive intra-operative and immediate post-operative hemorrhage. Thereafter, half or more of the initial loading dose should be re-administered every 12 h in order to maintain nadir factor levels greater than 50%. Factor activity should be measured every day and adjusted to maintain the desired level.

References

Björkman S, Carlsson M, Berntorp E (1994) Pharmacokinetics of factor IX in patients with haemophilia B. Methodological aspects and physiological interpretation. *Eur J Clin Pharmacol* **46**: 325–332.

Björkman S, Oh M, Spotts G, *et al.* (2012) Population pharmacokinetics of recombinant factor VIII: the relationships of pharmacokinetics to age and body weight. *Blood* **119**: 612–618.

Escobar MA (2010) Products used to treat haemophilia: dosing. In: Lee C, Hoots K, Berntop E (eds.), *Textbook of Haemophilia*. Blackwell Publishing.

Roberts HR, Escobar MA (2003) Other coagulation factor deficiencies. In: Loscalzo J, Schafer AI (eds.), *Thrombosis and Hemorrhage* (3rd edn.). Philadelphia: Lippincott Williams & Wilkins, pp. 575–598.

CASE STUDY 15

Compartment Syndrome

Miguel A. Escobar

Division of Hematology, University of Texas Health Science Center at Houston and Gulf States Hemophilia and Thrombophilia Center, Houston, TX, USA

A 32-year-old male with severe hemophilia A, without an inhibitor, tripped and fell on the stairs, injuring the left calf area. Since he "did not bleed into the knee" no factor infusion was administered. A few hours later he started to notice pain in the calf muscles but ignored it and continued his activities. About 8 h after the initial trauma he noticed an extensive induration of the calf with some tingling of his toes and decides to visit the emergency room. On examination his foot was swollen and there was discoloration of the toes. The calf was "rock hard" and very tender at palpation (Figure 15.1).

Q	How should the patient be managed?

The patient should have FVIII infused to raise the FVIII level to 100%, and a FVIII infusion at 4 units/kg/h should be started to maintain the FVIII level at 100%. Orthopedic surgery should see the patient emergently, and pressure readings in the various compartments of the calf should be measured. If the readings and the physical examination findings indicate the presence of compartment syndrome, fasciotomy should be performed emergently.

This patient underwent fasciotomies with the coverage of factor VIII. Luckily he had no sequelae from the event (Figure 15.2).

Compartment syndrome – Bleeding into a closed compartment muscle and tissue areas like hand, wrist, forearm, and anterior or posterior tibial compartments may result in the compression of nerves and blood vessels.

Hemophilia and Hemostasis: A Case-Based Approach to Management, Second Edition.
Edited by Alice D. Ma, Harold R. Roberts, Miguel A. Escobar.
© 2013 John Wiley & Sons, Ltd. Published 2013 by John Wiley & Sons, Ltd.

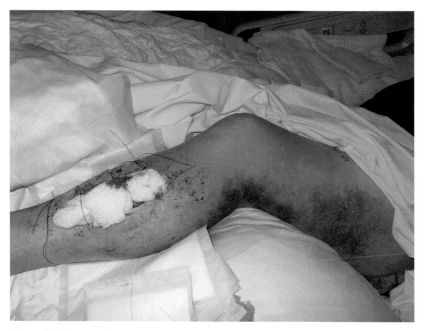

Figure 15.1 Severe hemophilia A patient with a compartment syndrome after trauma requiring fasciotomy.

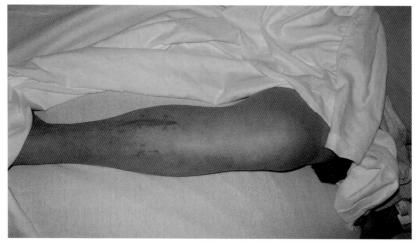

Figure 15.2 Satisfactory healing 3 months after fasciotomy.

Initial symptoms like pain and edema can be preceded by paresthesias and loss of distal pulses. In patients without hemophilia that develop a compartment syndrome, decompression with a fasciotomy is the treatment of choice. In hemophiliacs the management may be more conservative with aggressive factor replacement and frequent monitoring of pressures. Prompt treatment with replacement factor is indicated to maintain levels above 50% of normal. If replacement therapy fails to stop the progression, surgical decompression may be indicated.

References

Lancourt JE, Gilbert MS, Posner MA (1997) Management of bleeding and associated complications of hemophilia in the hand and forearm. *J Bone Joint Surg Am* **59**: 451–460.

Lintz F, Colombier JA, Letenneur J, Gouin F (2009) Management of long-term sequel of compartment syndrome involving the foot and ankle. *Foot Ankle Int* **30**: 847–853.

Llinás A, Silva M, Pasta G, *et al.* (2010) Controversial subjects in musculoskeletal care of haemophilia: cross fire. *Haemophilia* **16**: 132–135.

CASE STUDY 16

Successful Eradication of Factor VIII Inhibitor in Patient with Mild Hemophilia A Prior to Hemipelvectomy for Extensive Hemophilic Pseudotumor

Matthew Foster and Alice D. Ma
Division of Hematology/Oncology, University of North Carolina School of Medicine, Chapel Hill, NC, USA

A 69-year-old man with history of moderate hemophilia A, and baseline FVIII level of 3%, presented to the Hemophilia Treatment Center at the University of North Carolina for management of chronic swelling of the left thigh after being managed for years at a non-HTC center. The patient had a history of multiple traumatic injuries to both thighs, treated with FVIII. Six years prior, the patient had developed a "pathologic fracture" of the left femur with "bone cysts" noted. Malignancy was ruled out, and the patient underwent rod placement and was treated with bolus doses of FVIII for 1 week. One year later, the patient developed a re-fracture of the left thigh at the same site, which was again surgically repaired and treated with a week of bolus FVIII. Subsequently, the patient developed progressive swelling and pain in left thigh, necessitating complete bedrest. During this time, the patient also developed an inhibitor, with peak Bethesda titer of 40 BU, which was treated with intermittent rVIIa and prednisone. The patient has suffered significantly worsening swelling over past 2 years. His thigh had become so massive that he was bed bound at presentation.

One day after initial consultation at our hemophilia center, he presented to our emergency department with hemorrhage from a newly-formed sinus tract on his anterior left thigh (Figure 16.1). Factor VIII activity was 1%, and inhibitor titer was 1 BU. Imaging of the thigh and pelvis

Hemophilia and Hemostasis: A Case-Based Approach to Management, Second Edition.
Edited by Alice D. Ma, Harold R. Roberts, Miguel A. Escobar.
© 2013 John Wiley & Sons, Ltd. Published 2013 by John Wiley & Sons, Ltd.

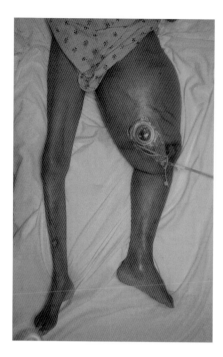

Figure 16.1 Pseudotumor at time of hospital admission. An ostomy bag with drain covers a bleeding sinus tract.

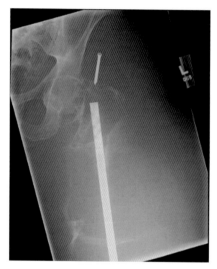

Figure 16.2 Plain film of the left femur showing osseous bone destruction, displaced intramedullary rod, and heterotopic ossification.

> **Q** How should the patient be managed at this point?

demonstrated massive hemophilic pseudotumor along the anterior and posterior surfaces of the iliac wing (Figure 16.2).

Acute bleeding was stabilized with rVIIa and red cell transfusion. He was treated with rituximab 375 mg/m², four doses given on days 1, 5, 12, and 19, in an attempt to eradicate his inhibitor prior to surgery. On day 19 (3 days

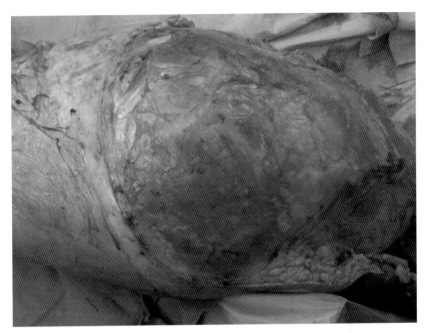

Figure 16.3 Intraoperative photograph showing hemipelvectomy specimen, with the cut surface of the pseudotumor.

pre-operatively) his inhibitor titer was 0 BU, and factor VIII activity 2%. Approximately 12 h pre-operatively he was treated with 100 units/kg recombinant factor VIII bolus followed by 6 units/kg/h continuous infusion, and was taken for left hemipelvectomy (Figure 16.3), hindquarter amputation and fasciocutaneous flap coverage. Estimated blood loss was 3 liters (including blood within the pseudotumor itself), and 7 units of packed red blood cells were transfused intra-operatively. Post-operatively he was maintained on recombinant factor VIII infusion, with factor VIII activity levels ranging from 84 to 187%. He required 2 units of packed red cells 2 days post-operatively, though no bleeding was apparent. No anamnestic inhibitor response occurred, and he was converted to bolus factor dosing upon transfer to a rehabilitation unit on the eighth post-operative day.

On the 22nd post-operative day, after 2 weeks of intensive rehabilitation, the patient was discharged home. At the time of discharge, he was able to transfer independently to his wheelchair (Figure 16.4), and was discharged to the care of his family.

Pseudotumors – Pseudotumors are rare complications of hemophilia with incidence among severe hemophilics of 1–2% (Magallón et al., 1994). They are usually triggered by intramuscular bleeding in the thigh or pelvis. These masses comprise cysts of serosanguinous material that expand over months to years, and may erode into bony or vascular structures. In retrospect, a pathologic fracture with bone cysts in a patient with hemophilia should have

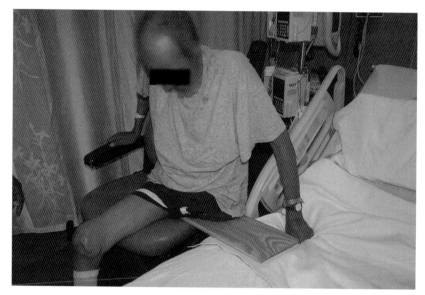

Figure 16.4 The patient transfers independently from bed to wheelchair after amputation and rehabilitation.

been assumed to have been a pseudotumor once a malignancy was ruled out. The patient should have received more prolonged, intensive therapy with factor replacement, and should have been seen sooner at an HTC.

When an inhibitor develops in cases of mild or moderate hemophilia, the clinical phenotype resembles that of patients with acquired hemophilia, with increased risk of soft tissue and gastrointestinal hemorrhage. Rituximab has been used successfully to eradicate inhibitors in cases of acquired hemophilia. More recently, this anti-CD20 monoclonal antibody has been shown in case series to eradicate inhibitors in mild and moderate congenital hemophilic patients (Dunkley *et al.*, 2006; Carcao *et al.*, 2006). Due to concerns of ongoing bleeding and risk of erosion into vascular structures, we accelerated rituximab dosing to allow for expedited operative intervention. The patient's inhibitor was successfully eradicated without a clinically significant anamnestic response.

References

Carcao M, St Louis J, Poon M-C, *et al.* (2006) Rituximab for congenital haemophiliacs with inhibitors: a Canadian experience. *Haemophilia* **12**: 7–18.

Dunkley S, Kershaw G, Young G, *et al.* (2006) Rituximab treatment of mild haemophilia A with inhibitors: a proposed treatment protocol. *Haemophilia* **12**: 663–667.

Magallón M, Monteagudo J, Altisent C, *et al.* (1994) Hemophilic pseudotumor: multicenter experience over a 25-year period. *Am J Hematol* **45**: 103–108.

Stasi R, Brunetti M, Stipa E, Amadori S. (2004) Selective b-cell depletion with rituximab for the treatment of patients with acquired hemophilia. *Blood* **103**: 4424–4428.

CASE STUDY 17

Coronary Artery Disease and Hemophilia

Alice D. Ma

Division of Hematology/Oncology, University of North Carolina, Chapel Hill, NC, USA

A 55-year-old man with severe hemophilia A without inhibitor presented with unstable angina. He was overweight with a BMI of 50. He had hypertension, type 2 diabetes mellitus, and hypercholesterolemia. He smoked 1 ppd and had done so for the past 40 years. His father had died of an MI at age 48. It was suspected that he had sleep apnea but had not undergone evaluation. He had chronic renal insufficiency with an estimated GFR of 40 mL/min. He had severe hemophilic arthopathy; he underwent right knee arthroplasty 2 years ago and left knee arthroplasty 6 months ago. He had pain in bilateral ankles, hips, and elbows for which he was on chronic narcotic therapy. He took recombinant FVIII on demand and had bleeds approximately 3–5 times monthly.

He has been resistant to the idea of prophylactic therapy because of relatively poor venous access due to body habitus and has developed exertional substernal chest burning. These episodes are increasing in frequency, and he developed rest pain last evening, lasting 2–4 minutes. The cardiology service wants to treat the patient with heparin and a GPIIbIIIa inhibitor, and do a cardiac catheterization.

Q1	How should this patient best be treated for his impending procedure?

Atherosclerotic heart disease is increasing in hemophilic patients as the population ages. While hemophilia was previously believed to confer protection against coronary artery disease, modern treatment with clotting

---

Hemophilia and Hemostasis: A Case-Based Approach to Management, Second Edition.
Edited by Alice D. Ma, Harold R. Roberts, Miguel A. Escobar.
© 2013 John Wiley & Sons, Ltd. Published 2013 by John Wiley & Sons, Ltd.

factor replacement, as well as the longer lifespans enjoyed by most hemophilics, has stripped this protection from our patients. This being said, there are no evidence-based guidelines to treat hemophilics with coronary artery disease, either on a chronic basis, or during procedures or acute coronary events. Practice guidelines such as those authored by Dr. Mannucci (2010) or Dr. Coppola (2010) suggest that factor replacement should be used to correct the hemostatic defect to normal, thus allowing anticoagulation and/or antiplatelet therapy.

During the acute period around his procedure, while heparin and a GPIIbIIIa inhibitor are used, the patient should be maintained at 80–100% FVIII activity levels, ideally via an initial bolus, followed by a continuous infusion. The continuous infusion eliminates the peaks and troughs seen with bolus dosing. Peak levels may be associated with thrombosis, and troughs increase the risk of bleeding, especially in someone being dually treated with heparin and a GPIIbIIIa inhibitor. FVIII activity levels should be checked at least daily, and infusion rates appropriately adjusted. For a simple catheterization, the patient should be maintained at 80–100% until 3–5 days after the procedure. This may be done using twice daily bolus dosing as an outpatient. Notably, measuring FVIII activity levels in a heparinized sample requires either heparin neutralization or sample dilution. In either case, the special coagulation laboratory should be notified to enable the appropriate measures to be taken to generate an accurate FVIII level. Lastly, if possible, catheterization should be done via a radial artery approach, which has been shown to minimize the bleeding risk.

Q2	What should be done if the patient requires stenting?

If the patient requires stenting, it is important to communicate with the cardiologists that a bare metal stent, rather than a drug-eluting stent, be used. The latter requires indefinite therapy with both clopidogrel as well as aspirin – a combination which then requires indefinite prophylactic factor treatment in a severe hemophilic. As above, FVIII levels should be kept at between 80 and 100% when the arterial puncture is performed, when the sheaths are removed, and when both heparin and a GPIIbIIIa inhibitor are being used. The use of closure devices to put more sustained pressure on the groin is preferred, unless the preferred radial artery approach is used. Again, measuring FVIII activity levels in a heparinized sample requires either heparin neutralization or sample dilution. In either case, the special coagulation laboratory should be notified to allow the appropriate measures to be taken to generate an accurate level.

After the stenting procedure, the patient should be kept on thrice weekly or qod prophylactic therapy with FVIII for the 1 to 3 months during which he will be on therapy with both clopidogrel and aspirin. After the clopidogrel is stopped, the prophylactic therapy may be weaned, with careful instruction to the patient to look for signs of bleeding. Any bleeding or drop in hemoglobin should be a cue to reinstitute factor prophylaxis at the original dose.

Q3	What if the patient requires CABG?

Careful coordination with the surgeon, anesthesia, the pump team as well as nursing, the coagulation laboratory, and the pharmacy needs to be done so that the surgical procedure and its aftermath go smoothly.

Pre-operatively, the patient should be bolused with 50 units/kg FVIII, followed immediately by institution of a FVIII continuous infusion at 4 units/kg/h. A stat FVIII level should be checked 30–60 min after the bolus, and only if it is above 80% should the patient be allowed to proceed to surgery.

It may be necessary to add FVIII to the fluid with which the pump is primed to ensure that the patient's FVIII is not diluted when the patient is placed on bypass. A FVIII level should be checked stat after the patient starts cardiopulmonary bypass (assuming the patient is not undergoing a CABG without bypass).

Post-operatively, another FVIII level should be checked and maintained at between 80 and 100%. Continuous infusion FVIII should be maintained for 7–10 days post-operatively, with levels maintained at 80–100%. Once the patient is discharged from hospital, we like the patient to treat himself with 50 units/kg daily to complete a 2-week course.

References

Coppola A, Tagliaferri A, Franchini M (2010) The management of cardiovascular diseases in patients with hemophilia. *Semin Thromb Hemost* **36**: 91–102.

Mannucci PM, Mauser-Bunschoten EP (2010) Cardiovascular disease in haemophilia patients: a contemporary issue. *Haemophilia* **16**(Suppl 3): 58–66.

CASE STUDY 18

Valve Replacement and Hemophilia

Alice D. Ma

Division of Hematology/Oncology, University of North Carolina, Chapel Hill, NC, USA

A 56-year-old man with a history of bicuspid aortic valve needs an aortic valve replacement. He has severe hemophilia A and no history of inhibitor. He had a right knee replacement 12 years ago without complications, and had been successfully treated for hepatitis C 5 years ago.

Q	How should he best be managed for his upcoming procedure?

Valvular heart surgery is currently the most common cardiac surgery performed on hemophilic patients. Typically, we recommend the use of tissue valves which obviate the necessity of long-term anticoagulation.

Careful coordination with the surgeon, anesthesia, the pump team as well as nursing, the coagulation laboratory, and the pharmacy needs to be done so that the surgical procedure and its aftermath go smoothly. Measuring FVIII activity levels in a heparinized sample requires either heparin neutralization or sample dilution. In either case, the special coagulation laboratory should be notified to enable the appropriate measures to be taken to generate an accurate level.

Pre-operatively, the patient should be bolused with 50 units/kg FVIII, followed immediately by institution of a FVIII continuous infusion at 4 units/kg/h. A stat FVIII level should be checked 30–60 min after the bolus, and only if it is above 80% should the patient be allowed to proceed to surgery.

It may be necessary to add FVIII to the fluid with which the pump is primed to ensure that the patient's FVIII is not diluted when he is placed

Hemophilia and Hemostasis: A Case-Based Approach to Management, Second Edition.
Edited by Alice D. Ma, Harold R. Roberts, Miguel A. Escobar.
© 2013 John Wiley & Sons, Ltd. Published 2013 by John Wiley & Sons, Ltd.

on bypass. A FVIII level should be checked stat after the patient starts cardiopulmonary bypass (assuming that the patient is not undergoing a CABG without bypass).

Post-operatively, another FVIII level should be checked and maintained at between 80 and 100%. Continuous infusion FVIII should be maintained for 7–10 days post-operatively, with levels maintained at 80–100%. During this time, the patient should be transitioned from unfractionated heparin to Coumadin. During the time the patient needs to be on Coumadin (usually 1–3 months), the patient should be maintained on strict qod prophylaxis to assure that the trough level remains above 30%. Careful coordination with the surgeons is required, since some surgeons do not mandate the use of anticoagulation.

References

Coppola A, Tagliaferri A, Franchini M (2010) The management of cardiovascular diseases in patients with hemophilia. *Semin Thromb Hemost* **36**: 91–102.

Mannucci PM, Mauser-Bunschoten EP (2010) Cardiovascular disease in haemophilia patients: a contemporary issue. *Haemophilia* **16**(Suppl 3): 58–66.

SECTION IV
Treatment for Other Conditions

Thyroid Biopsy and Hemophilia

Miguel A. Escobar

Division of Hematology, University of Texas Health Science Center at Houston and Gulf States
Hemophilia and Thrombophilia Center, Houston, TX, USA

A 32-year-old Hispanic male with a history of severe hemophilia A without
an inhibitor, and a thyroid nodule (Figure 19.1), underwent a thyroid
biopsy without the use of factor replacement therapy. Within an hour of
the procedure he started to experience a difficulty in breathing and a
swelling of the neck area. He returned to the hospital and was found to
have edema of the neck with dyspnea and odynophagia but no stridor and
some anxiety.

Q1	How should the patient be managed at this point?

This is a medical emergency. Factor VIII must be administered immediately
to raise his level to 100%. This should precede any imaging. The patient
received FVIII with improvement of the symptoms within 2h and fortu-
nately did not require intubation (Figure 19.2).

Discussion

Patients with coagulopathies and symptoms of upper airway obstruction
should be examined immediately. In patients with hemophilia, bleeding
from the floor of the mouth, pharynx or epiglottic area can result in partial
or complete airway obstruction. External compression of the airway due to
hemorrhage can also be seen after placement of neck or subclavian
catheters. Hence, such bleeding should be treated with aggressive
replacement of the deficient factor until complete resolution of the

Hemophilia and Hemostasis: A Case-Based Approach to Management, Second Edition.
Edited by Alice D. Ma, Harold R. Roberts, Miguel A. Escobar.
© 2013 John Wiley & Sons, Ltd. Published 2013 by John Wiley & Sons, Ltd.

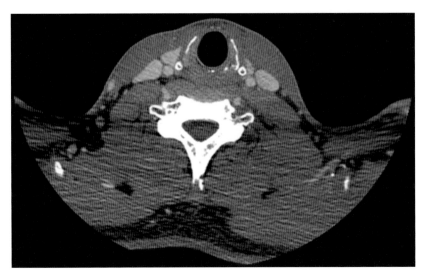

Figure 19.1 CT scan of the neck before biopsy.

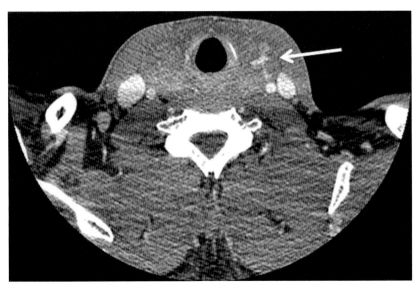

Figure 19.2 CT scan of the neck 2 h after thyroid biopsy without the coverage of FVIII. There is a diffuse enlargement of the thyroid gland involving both lobes and narrowing of the airway. In this image with contrast there is a focus of enhancement in the left lobe (arrow) which most likely corresponds to active bleeding.

bleeding is established. Doses to maintain factor levels above 80% should be the goal of treatment.

It is important to manage these patients with a multidisciplinary team that includes the ENT surgeons, hematologists and anesthesiologists. In some occasions prophylactic intubation may be necessary when the airway is closing to avoid the need for urgent airway rescue which can be sometimes difficult in the presence of edema. The airway can be assessed atraumatically via a transnasal flexible fiberoptic laryngoscopy prior to attempting endotracheal intubation. This approach will prevent unnecessary intubation in an inaccessible airway. Ultrasound is a non-invasive and inexpensive technique that can be used to monitor the hematoma.

Treatment with factor should be given daily for at least 7–10 days to ensure that there is adequate healing and no recurring hematoma.

References

Aspelin M, Petterson H, *et al.* (1984) Ultrasonographic examinations of muscle hematomas in hemophiliacs. *Acta Radiol Diagn* **25**: 513–516.

Jaryszak EM, Verghese ST, *et al.* (2010) Multidisciplany management of expanding bilateral neck hematomas in a patient with hemophilia A with high-titer inhibitor. *Int J Pediatr Otorhinolaryngol* **74**: 828–830.

CASE STUDY 20

Atrial Fibrillation and Bleeding Disorders

Alice D. Ma

Division of Hematology/Oncology, University of North Carolina, Chapel Hill, NC, USA

A 50-year-old man presented with a presyncopal event and was found to be in atrial fibrillation. He had a history of hypertension (on medication) and had recently been found to have a FXI activity level of <1%. He had no significant bleeding history, but nor had he had any significant bleeding challenges. He had never had surgery. He had had no tooth extractions, and no significant trauma. He denied easy bruising or prolonged bleeding with minor trauma.

He has had an echocardiogram showing a dilated left atrium without thrombus. The cardiologists would like to cardiovert him.

Q1	How should he be treated for his attempted cardioversion?

Conversion of atrial fibrillation (AF) to sinus rhythm is associated with a small incidence of embolic events, that may be due to either pre-existing or de novo thrombus formation. Anticoagulation reduces the incidence of embolization after cardioversion to less than 1% within 1 month.

However, this patient has a congenital bleeding disorder that may or may not be clinically significant. Patients with FXI deficiency have a spectrum of hemorrhagic phenotypes, with some patients having no bleeding, even with levels <1%, and some patients having significant bleeding with levels higher than 5%. This patient has no bleeding history, but has never been hemostatically challenged. We would therefore be conservative with treatment. For this reason, we would recommend that he should not receive antithrombotic therapy for AF that is <48 h in

---

Hemophilia and Hemostasis: A Case-Based Approach to Management, Second Edition.
Edited by Alice D. Ma, Harold R. Roberts, Miguel A. Escobar.
© 2013 John Wiley & Sons, Ltd. Published 2013 by John Wiley & Sons, Ltd.

duration. Should the AF persist past 48 h, we would recommend the use of either aspirin (81 mg) or clopidogrel (75 mg qd).

For his cardioversion, we would recommend the use of unfractionated heparin, while replacing FXI to >50% using FFP for 48 h. This may require plasma exchange to avoid giving the patient an excessive volume load.

Q2	How should patients with other bleeding disorders be treated for atrial fibrillation?

We would use the guidelines above, including replacing clotting factor, using concentrates when available, PCCs or plasma when concentrates are not available. We would maintain clotting factors replacement for the 48 h during which the patient is therapeutically anticoagulated. Long-term treatment with aspirin or clopidogrel for patients with persistent atrial fibrillation may require prophylactic factor replacement in cases of more severe bleeding disorders such as severe hemophilia A/B or type 3 VWD.

Reference

Mannucci PM, Mauser-Bunschoten EP (2010) Cardiovascular disease in haemophilia patients: a contemporary issue. *Haemophilia* **16**(Suppl 3): 58–66.

CASE STUDY 21

Chronic Upper Gastrointestinal Bleeding and Hemophilia

Alice D. Ma

Division of Hematology/Oncology, University of North Carolina, Chapel Hill, NC, USA

A 70-year-old man with mild hemophilia B, baseline FIX level of 12% presented with recurrent UGI bleeding due to GAVE syndrome (gastric antral vascular ectasia). On three separate occasions this year, he had had a 4–5 g drop in his hemoglobin value, associated with melena. These episodes were treated with FIX and red cell transfusions at his local hospital. He was referred to the HTC for further management. His past history is significant for hypertension, renal insufficiency with estimated GFR of 40 mL/min, congestive heart failure and degenerative joint disease, s/p bilateral hip replacements.

Q	What are options for management at this time?

Management of this complicated patient will require cooperation between both gastroenterology and the HTC. GAVE syndrome can be managed with sequential applications of laser photocoagulation. This will need to be done on a regular basis – especially around times of bleeding episodes. It is important to emphasize to the GI service that hemophilia alone does not account for the bleeding. Likewise, the HTC must assure the GI service that factor replacement will allow for any invasive procedure to be done without risk of abnormal bleeding.

Hemophilia and Hemostasis: A Case-Based Approach to Management, Second Edition.
Edited by Alice D. Ma, Harold R. Roberts, Miguel A. Escobar.
© 2013 John Wiley & Sons, Ltd. Published 2013 by John Wiley & Sons, Ltd.

The bleeding from GAVE syndrome can lead to chronic GI bleeding with iron deficiency anemia. This may require therapy, including iron replacement (parenteral therapy may be required on a chronic, regular basis) and periodic red cell transfusions.

A trial of prophylactic FIX replacement therapy may show benefit, but may also not be completely necessary.

CASE STUDY 22

Hematuria

Nidra Rodriguez

Division of Hematology, The University of Texas Health Science Center at Houston and Gulf States Hemophilia and Thrombophilia Center, Houston, TX, USA

A 45-year-old man with severe hemophilia B presented with recurrent episodes of asymptomatic hematuria.

> **Q** Are there any long-term sequelae of hematuria in patients with hemophilia?

The prevalence of hematuria in young adults ranges between 0.19 and 16.1% but it has been reported up to 21% in men over 50 years of age. However, in males with hemophilia, the prevalence has been reported as high as 66%. Even though the differential diagnosis for males with hematuria is broad, it has been typically considered to be benign in patients who have hemophilia. However, more recent data suggests that chronic and/or intermittent hematuria can be associated with an increased incidence of renal disease and a potentially increased risk of death secondary to renal disease. Therefore, it is important not to assume that hematuria is benign in all patients with hemophilia but rather to individualize each case and consider referral to a nephrologist, particularly if there is associated proteinuria, red blood cell casts, abnormal creatinine, and/or hypertension. In addition, there should be a low threshold for further evaluation in hemophilia patients who are infected with HIV and/or HCV.

References

Beck P, Evans KT (1972) Renal abnormalities in patients with haemophilia and Christmas disease. *Clin Radiol* **23**: 349–354.

Hemophilia and Hemostasis: A Case-Based Approach to Management, Second Edition. Edited by Alice D. Ma, Harold R. Roberts, Miguel A. Escobar.
© 2013 John Wiley & Sons, Ltd. Published 2013 by John Wiley & Sons, Ltd.

Kulkarni R, Soucie JM, Evatt B, *et al.* (2003) Renal disease among males with haemophilia. *Haemophilia* **9**: 703–710.

Messing EM, Young TB, Hunt VB, *et al.* (1992) Home screening for hematuria: results of a multiclinic study. *J Urol* **148**: 289–292.

Prentice CRM, Lindsay RM, Barr RD, *et al.* (1971) Renal complications in haemophilia and Christmas disease. *Q J Med* **40**: 47–61.

Soucie JM, Nuss R, Evatt B, *et al.* (2000) Mortality among males with hemophilia: relations with source of medical care. *Blood* **96**: 437–442.

Woolhandler S, Pels RJ, Bor DH, *et al.* (1989) Dipstick urinalysis screening of asymptomatic adults for urinary tract disorders. I. Hematuria and proteinuria. *JAMA* **262**: 1214–1219.

SECTION V
Other Issues in Hemophilia Care

CASE STUDY 23

Reproductive Options for Hemophilia A Carriers[*]

Kristy Lee

Department of Genetics, University of North Carolina School of Medicine, Chapel Hill, NC, USA

A 26-year-old female and her 27-year-old husband were seen during their 3-year-old son's clinic visit for severe hemophilia A. There was no family history of hemophilia (see Figure 23.1). They are interested in having additional children, but are concerned about the risk of having another child with this condition.

Q1	What is their risk of having another child with hemophilia?

Any female who has a son with hemophilia and no known family history of the condition begins with a 2 in 3, or 66%, chance of being a carrier. There is a 1 in 3, or 33%, chance that the child has hemophilia A due to a de novo mutation in the *F8* gene. However, by assessing the family history you may be able to further refine her risk of being a carrier by using Bayesian analysis. This will allow you to take into consideration if she has any unaffected brothers, uncles, nephews, or sons, which will decrease her *a priori* risk of being a carrier. In this family, the mother starts out with a 2/3 chance of being a carrier. However, if we take into consideration that she has two brothers that do not have hemophilia, we can reduce her chance of being a carrier to 1/3 by using Bayesian analysis (see Figure 23.2).

* The majority of the information presented would also be applicable to couples with a son with hemophilia B, with the exception of genetic testing recommendations.

Hemophilia and Hemostasis: A Case-Based Approach to Management, Second Edition.
Edited by Alice D. Ma, Harold R. Roberts, Miguel A. Escobar.
© 2013 John Wiley & Sons, Ltd. Published 2013 by John Wiley & Sons, Ltd.

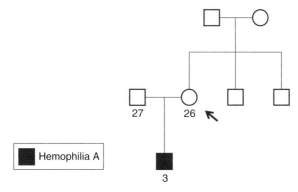

Figure 23.1 Pedigree illustrating patient with hemophilia and his family.

	Bayesian analysis	
	Mother is a carrier	Mother is not a carrier
Prior probability	2/3	1/3
Conditional probability (based on two unaffected brothers)	$(1/2)^2 = 1/4$	1
Joint probability	$2/3 \times 1/4 = 1/6$	$1/3 \times 1 = 1/3$
Posterior probability	$\dfrac{1/6}{1/6 + 1/3} = 1/3$	$\dfrac{1/3}{1/6 + 1/3} = 2/3$

Figure 23.2 Bayesian calculation to determine the mother's risk of being a carrier for hemophilia.

Since measuring FVIII activity levels can lead to false negative results in carrier females, the most informative way in which to test for carrier status is to order genetic testing to determine whether the woman has her son's mutation. If her son has not been genotyped, you would use the following algorithm for testing a male with severe hemophilia A:

1 intron 22 inversion analysis, if negative proceed
2 full sequencing of *F8* gene, if negative proceed
3 intron 1 inversion analysis, if negative proceed
4 *F8* gene duplication analysis

Molecular testing of the *F8* gene can detect mutations in greater than 98% of males with hemophilia A. Once the son's mutation is identified, you can test the mother to determine her carrier status. If genetic testing is unable to detect her son's mutation, you can inform your patient's mother that she is not a carrier for hemophilia. In this scenario, the risk of having a child with hemophilia is significantly reduced, but is not nil. A female with a previous child with hemophilia, who tests negative for her son's mutation, has a residual risk of having a child with hemophilia due to germline mosaicism. This phenomenon occurs when a portion of the female's egg cells harbor the *F8* gene mutation. The rate of germline mosaicism is somewhat higher in hemophilia A than in other X-linked conditions (but is certainly not as high as Duchenne Muscular Dystrophy, which has up to a 15% risk of mosaicism). Currently, there is no way to rule out the risk of germline mosaicism; therefore, a female with a previous child with hemophilia A and normal molecular testing for her son's *F8* gene mutation should be alerted to the small possibility of germline mosaicism. Unfortunately, exact risk numbers for germline mosaicism in hemophilia A are difficult to provide to couples. Couples concerned about the risk of germline mosaicism may wish to undergo prenatal diagnostic testing during a future pregnancy.

If the son's mutation is identified in the mother, this would confirm that she is a carrier for hemophilia.

Q2	What are the reproductive options to try to prevent or reduce the risk of having another child with this condition?

At this time, you can discuss reproductive options with the couple. There are options available during preconception and pregnancy. Preconception options include semen sorting and preimplantation genetic diagnosis (PGD). Prenatal testing options would include chorionic villus sampling (CVS) or amniocentesis followed by pregnancy termination of an affected fetus.

Semen sorting would be used in conjunction with intrauterine insemination (IUI) or in vitro fertilization (IVF) to attempt to conceive a female. A flow cytometer is used to sort the X chromosome spermatozoa from the Y chromosome spermatozoa. The goal is to put the couple's odds in favor of having a female child. While this technique is unable to prevent the daughter from being a carrier, it reduces the odds of having a son, who could inherit hemophilia. One facility in the United States offering semen sorting quotes a success rate as high as 88% in conceiving a female fetus. The couple choosing this option has to be comfortable with several issues. The couple will only be attempting to have a female child. The couple is still at risk of having a son with hemophilia, since the technique is not 100% successful. Finally, the couple must be comfortable using IUI or IVF in order to conceive a pregnancy.

PGD has a couple of advantages over semen sorting; however, it is also more costly. The cost of semen sorting is approximately 3,000 USD, while the cost of PGD is approximately 5,000 USD in addition to the costs associated with each cycle of IVF, which are approximately 15,000 USD per cycle. This technique is performed on embryos that have undergone IVF.

One cell is removed from the embryo to test for the known familial mutation. The embryos that have the *F8* mutation would not be used for pregnancy. This technique would allow the couple to have either a son or daughter, and it also has a higher success rate of preventing a son from having hemophilia. If there are additional embryos that do not have the mutation, these embryos can be frozen and used for future cycles of IFV or later pregnancies.

There are several barriers to preconception reproductive options. One significant barrier is cost. These procedures can be very costly and some health insurance companies do not cover, or have limited coverage, of the costs associated with these techniques. Even if medical costs are covered, or partially covered, there are ancillary costs involved, such as extensive travel costs associated with being seen at an institution equipped to provide these services.

Another significant barrier is ethical or religious beliefs. The couple may be uncomfortable with the idea of using these techniques to conceive a child. If the couple was considering PGD, they may also be concerned about the fate of the embryos that have inherited the familial mutation, or those that are not used for their pregnancy. These concerns must be addressed on an individual basis, and you may find in discussing these techniques that they are not good options for the couple.

If the couple had already conceived a pregnancy, genetic testing could be performed on a sample obtained via CVS around 10–12 weeks' gestation or an amniocentesis around 15–20 weeks' gestation to determine if the fetus was affected. Their only option to prevent having another child with hemophilia at that time would be to terminate the pregnancy.

References

Brower C, Thompson A. (2011) Hemophilia A. *Gene Reviews*. http://www.ncbi.nlm. nih.gov/books/NBK1404/. Accessed August 2011.

Genetic & IVF Institute (2011) *Genetic Services*. Accessed August 2011. http://www.givf. com/

Laurie AD, Hill AM, Harraway JR, *et al.* (2010) Preimplantation genetic diagnosis for hemophilia A using indirect linkage analysis and direct genotyping approaches. *J Thromb Haemost* **8**: 783–789.

Leuer M, Oldenburg J, Lavergne JM, *et al.* (2001) Somatic mosaicism in hemophilia A: a fairly common event. *Am J Hum Genet* **69**(1): 75–87.

Nussbaum R, McInnes R, Willard H. (2007) *Thompson and Thompson Genetics in Medicine* (7th edn.). Philadelphia: Saunders/Elsevier.

Zimmerman MA, Oldenburg J, Müller CR, Rost S (2010) Characterization of duplication breakpoints in the factor VIII gene. *J Thromb Haemost* **8**(12): 2696–2704.

CASE STUDY 24

Mild Hemophilia A with Discrepant FVIII Activity Levels

Alice D. Ma

Division of Hematology/Oncology, University of North Carolina, Chapel Hill, NC, USA

A 45-year-old man with a history of mild hemophilia A, baseline FVIII level of 20%, presented with severe neck and left arm pain, numbness, and need for paraspinal steroid injections.

His bleeding history is as follows: He presented at age 5 months with a forehead bruise after hitting his forehead. He had an aPTT which was quite prolonged and a factor VIII level was measured at 1.4%. Subsequent factor VIII levels ranged between 6 and 17%. At age 10 years, the patient developed left elbow hemarthrosis. He received no clotting factor, and his symptoms persisted for several weeks. At the age of 13, he had 2 right elbow bleeds. Seven years ago, the patient slipped at work and injured his right knee, which became swollen. He underwent arthroscopic surgery which led to further rebleeding and, overall, he received 18 doses of DDAVP but no clotting factor. The episode with his right knee continued to be troublesome for over a year with prolonged physical therapy and incomplete resolution to this day.

The patient also has a history of frank hematuria, requiring hospitalization at the ages of 13 and 15. He thinks he may have received clotting factor at that time. At the age of 12, he suffered a severe laceration on his right foot and may have received clotting factor. He also had a laceration of the left hand requiring 20 stitches and was treated with DDAVP.

Family history is remarkable for reported hemophilia in 4 maternal uncles, one of whom died from HIV. Two others have subsequently died, one from head trauma.

FVIII activity level measured by the one-stage assay is 20%. A FVIII activity level measured by the chromogenic method returns at 5%.

Hemophilia and Hemostasis: A Case-Based Approach to Management, Second Edition.
Edited by Alice D. Ma, Harold R. Roberts, Miguel A. Escobar.
© 2013 John Wiley & Sons, Ltd. Published 2013 by John Wiley & Sons, Ltd.

Q1	What is the biologic basis of this discrepancy in FVIII activity levels?

Patients and their families with mild/moderate hemophilia A and discrepant FVIII assays performed via the 1-stage and the chromogenic methods have been well described. Recently, a large population of mild/moderate French hemophilics from a single HTC was studied. 10% of patients were found to have discrepant results, with approximately 3% having chromogenic results higher than the 1-stage results, and 7% having lower chromogenic results than 1 stage assay results (similar to our patient). Patients with discrepant results can have lower FVIII chromogenic assay activities due to instability of the molecule with the more prolonged incubation required in the chromogenic assay. Mutations typically occur in the A1, A2, or A3 domains.

Q2	How should the patient be managed in the future?

This patient appears to behave more as if his "true" FVIII activity level is closer to the 5% reported by the chromogenic assay rather than the 20% given by the 1-stage assay. We recommend that the patient undergo DDAVP testing, with FVIII activity levels measured using the chromogenic method. This patient may require therapy with FVIII concentrates for more invasive procedures and severe trauma. Depending on the results of the DDAVP trial, he may be able to undergo paraspinal steroid injections with DDAVP coverage. Only if his FVIII activity level remains below 30% after therapy with DDAVP would we recommend pretreatment with FVIII concentrates prior to steroid injections.

References

Trossaërt M, Boisseau P, Quemener A, *et al.* (2011) Prevalence, biological phenotype and genotype in moderate/mild hemophilia A with discrepancy between one-stage and chromogenic factor VIII activity. *J Thromb Haemost* **9**: 524–530.

Bowyer AE, Goodeve A, Liesner R, *et al.* (2011) p.Tyr365Cys change in factor VIII: haemophilia A, but not as we know it. *Br J Haematol* **154**: 618–625.

SECTION VI
Compound Diagnoses

CASE STUDY 25

Hemophilia A with Tuberous Sclerosis and CNS Bleed

Alice D. Ma

Division of Hematology/Oncology, University of North Carolina, Chapel Hill, NC, USA

A 22-year-old man with severe hemophilia A and tuberous sclerosis presented with a large intracranial hemorrhage. Due to his tuberous sclerosis, he also had a history of renal insufficiency and angiomyolipomas of the kidney as well as a history of multiple ependymomas and a low-grade astrocytoma. There was no history of any inhibitor to FVIII.

Q1	How should the patient be managed acutely?

The patient should immediately be given a bolus of FVIII at 50 units/kg, followed immediately by institution of a continuous infusion of FVIII at 4 units/kg/h. A FVIII activity level should be checked 30–60 min after the bolus, as well as once or twice daily, and the patient should be rebolused and have the continuous infusion rate adjusted to maintain a FVIII activity level of around 100%. This level should be maintained for 3 weeks. At our institution, we would also add epsilon aminocaproic acid at 50 mg/kg given intravenously every 8 h for 2 weeks.

Additionally, since a massive intracranial hemorrhage can lead to a consumptive coagulopathy, the platelet count, fibrinogen, and PT/INR should be followed, and corrected with appropriate transfusions.

The patient made an astonishing recovery and was sent to a rehabilitation facility.

Hemophilia and Hemostasis: A Case-Based Approach to Management, Second Edition.
Edited by Alice D. Ma, Harold R. Roberts, Miguel A. Escobar.
© 2013 John Wiley & Sons, Ltd. Published 2013 by John Wiley & Sons, Ltd.

Q2	How should this patient be managed chronically?

Given that the patient has tuberous sclerosis with underlying ependymomata, he remains at high risk for recurrent intracranial hemorrhage. We would therefore recommend that the patient be maintained on prophylactic FVIII infusions given qod indefinitely. Additionally, the patient must maintain superb control of his blood pressure.

CASE STUDY 26

Familial Risk Assessment for Individuals with Hemophilia A and von Willebrand Disease

Kristy Lee

Department of Genetics, University of North Carolina School of Medicine, Chapel Hill, NC, USA

A 15-year-old male and his 12-year-old brother with severe hemophilia A were seen to establish care at their local Comprehensive Hemophilia Clinic after their family's recent relocation to the area. As part of their initial consultation, a three-generation pedigree was drawn. Of note, their mother reported that her father had a diagnosis of hemophilia A. Also of note, the boys' father reported a history of epistaxis, easy bruising, and excessive bleeding after his wisdom teeth extraction in his 20s. He also reported a brother with epistaxis as a child. Based on this family history, the clinician was concerned about the possibility that the father could have von Willebrand disease (VWD). During this visit, the clinician obtained a blood sample from the father to evaluate him for VWD, and his results from biochemical testing indicate that he has VWD type 1. The complete pedigree is shown below (see Figures 26.1 and 26.2).

Q	What is the risk of each of these conditions for relatives, including parents, siblings and children, and what is the recommended genetic work up for these family members?

With two relatively common genetic conditions, it is not surprising to observe a subset of the bleeding disorder population with hemophilia and VWD in the same family. However, a patient having of family history of two genetic conditions can certainly complicate accurate risk assessment.

Hemophilia and Hemostasis: A Case-Based Approach to Management, Second Edition.
Edited by Alice D. Ma, Harold R. Roberts, Miguel A. Escobar.
© 2013 John Wiley & Sons, Ltd. Published 2013 by John Wiley & Sons, Ltd.

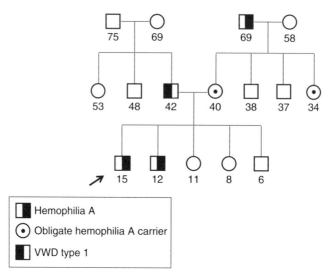

Figure 26.1 Pedigree illustrating the patients with hemophilia and their family history.

In this setting, the clinician must consider the risk of each of these conditions for each relative separately.

VWD type 1 is inherited in an autosomal dominant fashion. Therefore, the patients with hemophilia and their three other siblings each have a 50% risk of having inherited VWD. Since the de novo mutation rate in the VWF gene is unknown, we have to assume that each of the father's siblings and his parents also have up to a 50% chance of to have inherited a mutation in the *VWF* gene. We would recommend that each of these relatives have an evaluation to determine whether or not they have VWD.

In many clinics, a standard biochemical work up for VWD disease is usually performed in lieu of or in addition to molecular testing of the *VWF* gene. However, in the setting of a family history of hemophilia A using molecular testing of the *VWF* gene to complement the biochemical work up should be considered. The *VWF* gene is currently thought to be the only gene associated with VWD; however, it is plausible that an additional gene(s) will be associated with this condition in the future. Full sequencing of the *VWF* gene is thought to identify a mutation in ~65% of individuals with a diagnosis of VWD type 1. If the full sequencing analysis is normal, a dosage assay can be ordered to look for a partial or complete gene deletion or duplication. It is unclear at this time what proportion of individuals with VWD type 1 have a gene deletion or duplication mutation.

Given that not every individual with VWD has an identifiable mutation, it is best to begin genetic testing in an individual with a biochemical diagnosis of this condition. In this family, genetic testing was initiated in the father, who now had a biochemical diagnosis of this condition.

His testing was able to identify a mutation in the *VWF* gene, which was denoted as VWF c.3614G>A (p.R1205H). Each of the children and his brother were tested for this mutation. The mutation was identified in his 15 year son with hemophilia, his 6 year old son and his brother. Since this condition is not completely penetrant, it is always important to correlate the molecular test results with biochemical testing for VWD.

Based on the family history of hemophilia A in the children's maternal grandfather, we know that their mother and maternal aunt are obligate carriers for hemophilia, since hemophilia A is an X-linked condition. This informs us that the two daughters each have a 50% chance of being carriers for hemophilia. Measuring factor VIII to determine carrier status is not recommended in most situations; due to the fact that females who are carriers for hemophilia A can have factor VIII levels in the normal range. Therefore, molecular testing of the *F8* gene is recommended. The majority of mutations associated with hemophilia A can be detected via current molecular testing. However, it is still recommend that genetic testing be initiated in a male with hemophilia to ensure that the familial mutation can be detected. This allows female relatives to have informative carrier testing.

In this family, molecular testing was initiated in the 15 year old son with hemophilia, and he was found to have the intron 22 inversion. This result allowed us the opportunity to offer testing to his two sisters. The optimal age to offer carrier testing for hemophilia A is still somewhat under debate. We typically wait to offer carrier testing to at risk females until young adulthood or later in the teenage years, unless the child is experiencing bleeding symptoms or the parents wish to have the testing performed at an earlier age. This allows the child to make an informed decision when they are older regarding whether or not they are interested in pursuing carrier testing. However, in the setting of a family history of two bleeding disorders the decision was to proceed with carrier testing in both daughters. The 11 year old daughter was found to carry the intron 22 inversion, and the 8 year old daughter does not carry this mutation.

After completing the risk assessment and genetic testing for immediate family members for hemophilia A and VWD, we determined that the father, maternal uncle, 15 year old son and 6 year old son have VWD. Therefore, we determine that the 15 year old son not only has hemophilia A, but he also has VWD. We also determined that the 11 year daughter is a carrier for hemophilia, but does not have VWD. Finally, we were able to determine that the 8 year daughter is not a carrier for hemophilia and does not have VWD. To our knowledge the father's parents and sister have yet to be evaluated for VWD, but the family has alerted them to their risk of also having a diagnosis of VWD. The updated pedigree is below (see

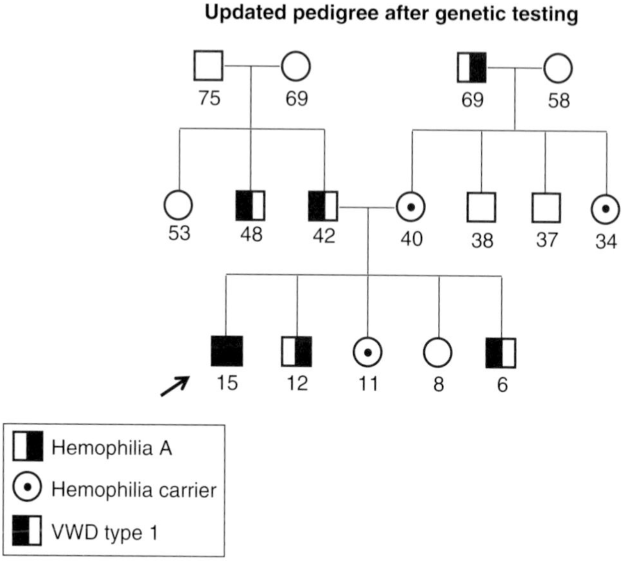

Updated pedigree after genetic testing

Figure 26.2 Pedigree illustrating the patients with hemophilia and their updated family history after additional genetic testing for hemophilia A and VWD was performed.

Figure 26.2). An accurate risk assessment is vital to identify at risk relatives and diagnose them properly.

References

Brower C, Thompson A. Hemophilia A. *Gene Reviews*. Accessed January 2012. http://www.ncbi.nlm.nih.gov/books/NBK1404/

Goodeve A, James P. von Willebrand Disease. *Gene Reviews*. Accessed January 2012. http://www.ncbi.nlm.nih.gov/books/NBK7014/

James P, Di Paola J. The application of genetics to inherited bleeding disorders. *Haemophilia*. 2010 Jul; **16** Suppl 5: 35–39.

Keeney S, Cumming AM. The molecular biology of von Willebrand disease. *Clin. Lab. Haem.* 2001; **23**: 209–230.

Nussbaum R, McInnes R, Willard H. (2007) *Thompson and Thompson Genetics in Medicine.* (7th ed.) Philadelphia: Saunders/Elsevier.

CASE STUDY 27

Hemophilia A and Hereditary Hemorrhagic Telangiectasia

Raj Sundar Kasthuri

Division of Hematology/Oncology, University of North Carolina School of Medicine, Chapel Hill, NC, USA

The patient is a 54-year-old African-American man with hemophilia A. He was diagnosed with severe hemophilia A at the age of 6 months. He does not have history of a factor VIII inhibitor. Comorbidities include HIV, hepatitis C, and hemophilic arthropathy. Of note, the patient also has a history of epistaxis that has progressively worsened with age. He has been on factor VIII prophylaxis 3 times a week for many years to help with the epistaxis. About 6 years ago, his hematologist pursued evaluation for a coexisting bleeding diathesis, such as von Willebrand disease, and this work-up was negative. As epistaxis was the primary symptom and as the patient's father reportedly had similar symptoms of epistaxis, the possibility of hereditary hemorrhagic helangiectasia (HHT) was raised. The patient was referred to ENT and fiberoptic endoscopy revealed numerous mucocutaneous telangiestasias in the nasal cavity, a few telangiectasias in the mouth and lips, and a diagnosis of HHT was made.

Q1	What is HHT and how does one manage epistaxis associated with HHT?

HHT or Osler–Weber–Rendu syndrome is an inherited disorder characterized by the abnormal development of blood vessels resulting in mucocutaneous telagiectasias and visceral arterial-venous malformations (AVMs). Mucocutaneous telangiectasias primarily involve the nose, mouth, lips, and fingers although telangiectasias can also be present over other areas. AVMs predominantly develop in the lungs, brain, and gastrointestinal

Hemophilia and Hemostasis: A Case-Based Approach to Management, Second Edition.
Edited by Alice D. Ma, Harold R. Roberts, Miguel A. Escobar.
© 2013 John Wiley & Sons, Ltd. Published 2013 by John Wiley & Sons, Ltd.

tract. Overall, HHT is a debilitating disorder with a significant impact on the quality of life in affected individuals.

The estimated prevalence of HHT is 1:5,000. Thus there are approximately 60,000 affected individuals in the USA and 1.4 million people affected world wide. HHT has an autosomal dominant inheritance. It is characterized by phenotypic heterogeneity resulting in varying disease severity among affected individuals within the same family. Mutations in the genes encoding two proteins, endoglin (ENG) and activin receptor-like kinase-1 (ACVRL-1 or ALK-1), account for 75–80% of HHT. In addition, mutations in the MADH4 gene (encoding for SMAD-4) are associated with a syndrome of juvenile polyposis and HHT. Genetic testing for these mutations is available.

The most common clinical feature of HHT is the presence of mucocutaneous telangiectasias, which are present in over 90% of affected individuals by adulthood. About 90–95% of affected individuals also develop varying degrees of epistaxis from bleeding telangiectasias during their lifetime. Pulmonary AVMs (PAVMs) develop in 30–50% of affected individuals and are associated with the risk for massive hemoptysis, hemothorax, paradoxical embolism, and brain abscesses. Intracranial AVMs (CAVMs) occur in 5–10% of affected individuals and confer a risk for hemorrhagic stroke, seizures, and death. Telangiectasias in the GI tract develop with increasing age and are seldom noted in patients under 40 years of age. These can lead to chronic GI blood loss in about 25% of affected individuals. AVMs in the liver are commonly seen in older patients with HHT, although only a minority of these are large enough to result in the development of shunts and associated complications, such as biliary necrosis or cardiac failure.

The diagnosis of HHT is made mainly on clinical grounds as guided by the Curacao diagnostic criteria. These comprise four criteria: (a) history of chronic and persistent epistaxis; (b) presence of mucocutaneous telangiectasias; (c) presence of visceral AVMs; and (d) family history of HHT in a first-degree relative. The presence of three or more criteria makes a definitive diagnosis of HHT while ≤1 criterion makes HHT unlikely. Genetic testing is also available and is generally used to identify the familial mutation in the proband so that other at-risk individuals in the family can be tested for HHT. Of note, it is estimated that only ~10% of individuals with HHT carry the diagnosis and the vast majority of affected individuals are as yet undiagnosed.

Early diagnosis of HHT can significantly impact the morbidity and mortality associated with this disorder. Current guidelines recommend screening for visceral AVMs in all patients with HHT with the goal of early detection and intervention to prevent complications. Along these lines, screening for PAVMs should be pursued at the time of diagnosis of HHT.

This can be performed using echocardiography with saline contrast or chest CT scan. If echocardiography is pursued, it is important for the performing technician/physician to be aware that PAVMs are associated with delayed appearance of saline contrast in the left heart as opposed to early appearance of contrast in patients with a patent foramen ovale. If the echocardiogram is positive, a chest CT will be necessary to identify the location and size of the PAVM(s). If screening does not reveal the presence of PAVMs, it should be repeated every 3–5 years because affected individuals can develop new PAVMs over time. Screening for CAVMs should also be pursued at the time of diagnosis. This should be done with an MRI/MRA scan of the brain. Unlike PAVMs, it is believed that affected individuals do not develop new CAVMs during their lifetime. Therefore, if initial screening is negative, no further screening for CAVMs is needed. If the initial screening for CAVMs is performed in childhood, a repeat MRI/MRA after age 18 should be considered. Screening for GI or liver AVMs in the asymptomatic patient is not currently recommended.

Q2	What additional measures need to be instituted in a patient with severe hemophilia A and HHT?

The management of a patient with HHT involves the following:

a. *Treatment of epistaxis.* All patients should be educated on techniques for prevention and self-management in cases of mild-moderate epistaxis. These involve use of humidifiers, avoiding medications like aspirin or NSAIDS, use of saline nasal sprays or application of vaseline or saline gels to the nostrils, nasal packing at times of epistaxis, etc. In patients with frequent and moderate/severe epistaxis, additional measures will be necessary. A number of these approaches are not approved indications for the medications used and this should be discussed with the patients. Topical estrogen-based ointments and antifibrinolytic agents can be effective in patients with moderate epistaxis. There are also reports on the successful use of tamoxifen, thalidomide, and bevacizumab in the treatment of severe epistaxis in patients with HHT. Invasive procedures such as cauterization of telangiectasias should be used as an adjunct to medical therapy, which should be the mainstay of treatment. If medical approaches are ineffective, surgery may be necessary to control epistaxis and septodermatoplasty may be considered.

b. *Management of iron deficiency and anemia.* Iron deficiency anemia is often inadequately treated in patients with HHT. Aggressive iron replacement is often necessary in order to keep up with the ongoing blood loss in these patients. Along these lines, if oral iron replacement is not successful in correcting the iron deficiency (either because of intolerance to oral iron or excessive bleeding), intravenous iron replacement should be pursued. Patients may also require supportive transfusions.

c. *Management of visceral AVMs.* Recommendations on screening for visceral AVMs have already been discussed. The treatment of visceral AVMs primarily involves embolization. PAVMs with a feeding artery diameter larger than 0.2–0.3 mm should be embolized. This is primarily done by interventional radiology. Similarly, embolization or other measures like cyber-knife radiation should be considered in case of CAVMs that are deemed to confer significant risk. Smaller AVMs are generally followed with repeated imaging studies. In general, cauterization is not believed to be a useful approach for the management of GI telangiectasias as the lesions tend to recur with time. Therefore, such invasive procedures should be used primarily as an adjunct. Patients with symptomatic liver AVMs are difficult to manage, and embolization is often not a viable approach in these cases. Recent reports have shown good results with the use of bevacizumab in patients with liver AVMs and liver transplant may be indicated in severe cases with liver failure.

d. *Genetic counseling for affected individuals and family members.* This is a very important component of the care of patients/families with HHT. At-risk family members must be identified, evaluated, and tested. All patients with HHT should receive genetic counseling and a genetics counselor should be involved, where possible.

e. *Dental prophylaxis.* Institution of antibiotic prophylaxis before dental procedures is essential in patient with HHT.

f. Finally, given the complicated and multidisciplinary approach to the care of patients with HHT, it is recommended that patients with HHT be managed under the guidance of HHT Centers of Excellence. There are currently 12 HHT Centers of Excellence in the USA and a number of Centers world wide (www.hht.org).

Treatment of epistaxis in the patient with severe hemophilia

Management of HHT-associated epistaxis in the patients with severe hemophilia can be very challenging. It is essential to adequately treat the hemophilia component with institution of factor prophylaxis, as was pursued in this patient. Depending on the severity of the epistaxis, simple measures such as use of humidifiers and nasal moisturizers may be inadequate in these patients. Use of an estrogen-based ointment applied to the nasal mucosal twice daily can be helpful in mild–moderate cases. Antifibrinolytic agents or other anti-angiogenic drugs like thalidomide or bevacizumab may be necessary in severe cases. Cauterization of bleeding telangiectasias is a useful stop-gap measure but is not a long-term solution in HHT-associated epistaxis. If all of the above measures fail, surgery such as septodermatoplasty should be considered.

In the case of the patient discussed above, he is currently on three times weekly factor VIII for prophylaxis, amicar 3 g three times daily (off-label use) and was started on thalidomide (off-label use) 3 months ago. He reports improvement in the frequency and severity of epistaxis but continues to have episodes 2–3 times a week. He also receives intravenous iron every 3–4 months as he does not tolerate oral iron.

References

Dupuis-Girod S, Bailly S, Plauchu H (2010) Hereditary hemorrhagic telangiectasia: from molecular biology to patient care. *J Thromb Haemost* **8**: 1447–1456.

Faughnan ME, Palda VA, Garcia-Tsao G, *et al.* (2011) International guidelines for the diagnosis and management of hereditary haemorrhagic telangiectasia. *J Med Genet* **48**: 73–87.

Karnezis TT, Davidson TM (2011) Efficacy of intranasal Bevacizumab (Avastin) treatment in patients with hereditary hemorrhagic telangiectasia-associated epistaxis. *Laryngoscope* **121**: 636–638.

Lebrin F, Srun S, Raymond K, *et al.* (2010) Thalidomide stimulates vessel maturation and reduces epistaxis in individuals with hereditary hemorrhagic telangiectasia. *Nat Med* **16**: 420–428.

Mitchell A, Adams LA, MacQuillan G, *et al.* (2008) Bevacizumab reverses need for liver transplantation in hereditary hemorrhagic telangiectasia. *Liver Transpl* **14**: 210–213.

PART II
von Willebrand Disease

Management during Procedures

CASE STUDY 28

Type 1 von Willebrand Disease and Tonsillectomy

Trinh T. Nguyen[1] and Miguel A. Escobar[2]

[1] Division of Hematology, University of Texas Health Science Center at Houston

[2] Gulf States Hemophilia and Thrombophilia Center, Houston, TX, USA

A 12-year-old Hispanic female with type 1 von Willebrand disease (VWD) required tonsillectomy and adenoidectomy for recurrent tonsillitis. Baseline laboratory studies: factor VIII 23%; VWF antigen was 45%; VWF ristocetin cofactor assay was 36%

Q	How should this patient be optimally managed?

The management of patients with type 1 VWD undergoing minor surgery in the upper airway includes prophylaxis with hemostatic agents such as antifibrinolytics, desmopressin (DDAVP), and/or von Willebrand factor (VWF) concentrates. A dose of an antifibrinolytic agent such as tranexamic acid or aminocaproic acid should be administered prior to surgery and continued PO every 6 h post-operatively when the patient is able to tolerate oral intake. Duration of therapy would be at least 5–10 days to prevent delayed bleeding. If the patient is known to have an adequate response to DDAVP, a dose should be administered prior to the procedure. The recommended dosing is 150 mcg/spray intra nasally in one nostril if the patient weighs less than 50 kg and 1 spray per nostril if the patient's weight is greater than 50 kg (total dose 300 mcg). Desmopressin can be continued daily×three doses in addition to the scheduled antifibrinolytic agent. If the patient is known to be a poor responder to DDAVP, then plasma-derived VWF concentrate may be used with goal VWF:RCo level 30–50 IU/dL for at least 1–3 days. The dosing recommendation consists of a prophylactic loading dose of 30–60 units/kg (in VWF:RCO IU/kg) followed

Hemophilia and Hemostasis: A Case-Based Approach to Management, Second Edition.
Edited by Alice D. Ma, Harold R. Roberts, Miguel A. Escobar.
© 2013 John Wiley & Sons, Ltd. Published 2013 by John Wiley & Sons, Ltd.

by 20–40 units/kg every 12–48 h thereafter. Other local agents such a topical thrombin and fibrin sealants are also options to help achieve local hemostasis.

This patient received a dose of aminocaproic acid pre-operatively. She was not a responder to DDAVP; thus, she received a dose of VWF concentrate 30 min prior to the procedure. Post-operatively, she was admitted to the 23-h observation unit and received a second and third dose of VWF concentrate 12 and 24 h after the first dose in addition to the scheduled antifibrinolytics. At discharge, she completed 10 days total of therapy with aminocaproic acid without bleeding complications.

Reference

US Department of Health and Human Services, National Institutes of Health, National Heart and Lung and Blood Institute Full Report on: *The Diagnosis, Evaluation, and Management of von Willebrand Disease*, December 2007. NIH Publication No. 08-5832.

CASE STUDY 29

von Willebrand Disease and Dental Surgery

Trinh T. Nguyen[1] and Miguel A. Escobar[2]

[1]Division of Hematology, University of Texas Health Science Center at Houston

[2]Gulf States Hemophilia and Thrombophilia Center, Houston, TX, USA

A 17-year-old WM with type 1 von Willebrand disease (VWD) required dental surgery for unerupted mandibular 3rd molars.

Q1	What is the optimal management of type 1 VWD patients undergoing dental procedures?

The management of patients with type 1 VWD undergoing minor surgeries in the upper airway includes prophylaxis with hemostatic agents such as antifibrinolytics, DDAVP, and/or von Willebrand factor (VWF) concentrates. A dose of antifibrinolytic therapy (Table 29.1) should be administered prior to surgery and continued PO every 6–8 h post-operatively when the patient is able to tolerate oral intake. Duration of therapy should be at least 5–10 days to prevent delayed bleeding. If the patient is known to have an adequate response to DDAVP (Table 29.2), a dose should be administered prior to the procedure. The recommended dosing is 150 mcg/spray intra-nasally in one nostril if the patient weighs less than 50 kg and one spray per nostril if the patient's weight is greater than 50 kg (total dose 300 mcg). Another option is intravenous DDAVP at 0.3 mcg/kg/dose. Desmopressin can be continued daily×three doses in addition to a scheduled antifibrinolytic agent. If the patient is known to be a poor responder to DDAVP, plasma-derived VWF concentrates may be used with goal VWF:RCo level 30–50 IU/dL for at least 1–3 days. The recommended dosing consists of a prophylactic loading dose of 30–60 units/kg (in VWF:RCO IU/kg) followed by 20–40 units/kg every 12–48 h thereafter.

Hemophilia and Hemostasis: A Case-Based Approach to Management, Second Edition.
Edited by Alice D. Ma, Harold R. Roberts, Miguel A. Escobar.
© 2013 John Wiley & Sons, Ltd. Published 2013 by John Wiley & Sons, Ltd.

Table 29.1 Antifibrinolytic dosage and routes of administration – dosing variable between studies.

Antifibrinolytic *one dose 1 hour prior to procedure	Route: Oral (swish and swallow or swish and spit)	Route: IV
	Adults: 4–6 g PO q 4–6 h×5–7 days or until hemostasis achieved	Adults: 4–5 g IV loading dose; Then 4–5 g IV q 4–6 hours×5–7 days or until hemostasis achieved
Aminocaproic acid	Pediatrics: 25–100 mg/kg/dose PO q 4–6 hours×5–7 days or until hemostasis achieved	Pediatrics: 50–100 mg/kg/dose IV q 4–6 hours×5–7 days or until hemostasis achieved
	Or 25% mouthwash four times a day×5–7 days	
Tranexamic acid	Adults: 1,300 gram PO q8 h×2–8 days Pediatrics: 10–15 mg/kg PO q 8 h×2–8 days Or 5–10% mouthwash 10 mL PO four times a day	Adults/Pediatrics: 10–15 mg/kg IV q 8 h×2–8 days

Table 29.2 Desmopressin challenge results.

	Factor VIII (%)	VWF:Ag (%)	VWF:RCo (%)
Pre-DDAVP	7	23	15
Two hours post DDAVP	36	106	97
Increase by	Five-fold	Five-fold	Six-fold

Other local agents such a topical thrombin and fibrin sealants are also options to help to achieve local hemostasis.

Q2	What is considered a good response to DDAVP?

In this patient, a DDAVP challenge was done prior to his surgery (Table 29.2). A good response to DDAVP shows a two- to five-fold increase in factor VIII and VWF antigen level and functional assay. Our patient was admitted for 23-h observation. Pre-operatively, he received a dose of aminocaproic acid and one spray per nostril of DDAVP 1 h prior to surgery. Post-operatively, he received another two 24-h daily doses of DDAVP and 10 days total of antifibrinolytic therapy without bleeding complications. He did not require von Willebrand factor concentrate to achieve hemostasis.

References

Brewer A, Correa ME (2006) *Guidelines for Dental Treatment of Patients with Inherited Bleeding Disorders*. Treatment of Hemophilia Monograph No. 40, World Federation of Hemophilia.

Mannucci PM (1998) Hemostatic drugs. *N Engl J Med* **339**(4): 245–253.

Nitu-Whalley IC, *et al.* (2001) Retrospective review of the management of elective surgery with desmopressin and clotting factor concentrates in patients with von Willebrand disease. *Am J Hematol* **66**(4): 280–284.

Shah SB, *et al.* (1998) Perioperative management of von Willebrand's disease in otolaryngologic surgery. *Laryngoscope* **108**(1 Pt 1): 32–36.

US Department of Health and Human Services, National Institutes of Health, National Heart and Lung and Blood Institute Full Report on: *The Diagnosis, Evaluation, and Management of von Willebrand disease*, December 2007. NIH Publication No. 08-5832.

CASE STUDY 30

von Willebrand Disease and Gastrointestinal Surgery

Marshall Mazepa and Alice D. Ma

Division of Hematology/Oncology, University of North Carolina, Chapel Hill, NC, USA

An otherwise healthy 45-year-old woman with severe type 1 von Willebrand disease (VWD) presented with chronic cholestasis which required an elective cholecystectomy. Her pre-operative VWD assays were as follows: VWF Antigen (VWF:Ag) 25 IU/dL; VWF Activity (VWF:RCo) 22 IU/dL; (factor VIII carrier activity) FVIII:C 33 IU/dL. She had never undergone a DDAVP trial.

Q	How should the patient be managed for this surgery?

The treatment strategy for VWD may employ the use of one or several approaches: (1) increase the endogenous circulating VWF and FVIII:C with the use of desmopressin (DDAVP); (2) increase the circulating VWF and FVIII:C from exogenous, plasma-derived, virally activated concentrates; and (3) use of agents whose action is not directly on VWF or FVIII, but rather hemostasis through alternative targets (most commonly being antifibrinolytic therapy).

Guidelines for surgical prophylaxis have recently been published for evidenced-based decision making for the management of VWD, and offer guidance for the diagnosis and management of VWD (Nichols *et al.*, 2008). Factors to consider when making a treatment strategy include the patient's subtype of VWD and responsiveness to desmopressin, type of surgery (major, minor, or simple minor procedures), and comorbid conditions. Use of von Willebrand factor/factor VIII concentrate is recommended for type 2B, type 3, and all desmopressin-unresponsive cases. Thus, for patients

Hemophilia and Hemostasis: A Case-Based Approach to Management, Second Edition.
Edited by Alice D. Ma, Harold R. Roberts, Miguel A. Escobar.
© 2013 John Wiley & Sons, Ltd. Published 2013 by John Wiley & Sons, Ltd.

with severe type 1 VWD, a trial of DDAVP responsiveness may be of some utility, particularly for those patients without cardiovascular disease and in whom the procedure requires fewer days of hemostasis. A DDAVP challenge is administered IV (0.3 mcg/kg) or inhaled (Stimate), however IV administration is preferred for prophylaxis of surgical bleeding and is our practice. Caution should be taken particularly in the elderly due to risk of hyponatremia and cardiovascular disease (due to rare reports of myocardial infarction associated with DDAVP administration). Plasma-derived, virally inactivated concentrates may be used in addition to, or in place of, desmopressin for major surgery. The type of surgery (major, minor) dictates the target number of days of VWF replacement; cholecystectomy is listed as a major surgery for the previously noted guidelines, requiring 7–14 days of replacement. Humate-P ® (CSL Behring, Marburg, Germany) is the plasma-derived product used at our facility, and requires an initial loading dose (goal VWF:RCo 100 IU/dL for major surgery) followed by maintenance doses (days 1–3 goal VWF:RCo ≥ 50 IU/dL; days 4–14 goal VWF:RCo ≥ 30 IU/dL) (Nichols et al., 2008; Gill et al., 2011).

Our practice has been to use a VWF-containing FVIII concentrate given with an initial loading dose of 50–60 RCo units/kg given 30–60 min prior to surgery. We give further doses of 40–60 RCo units/kg every 12 h for a further two doses, then follow with 40–60 RCo units/kg every 24 h to complete 5–7 post-operative days. If the patient has been shown to be responsive to DDAVP, then Stimate nasal spray could be used at one squirt in each nostril on post-operative days 8–10.

Concern has also been raised about the risk for thrombosis in the post-operative period, especially in the setting of elevated FVIII:C levels. Recommendations by the NHLBI guidelines include monitoring both a VWF:RCo and FVIII:C at least once daily during days 1–7 post-operatively. Given the risk of thrombosis, it is also not recommended to exceed VWF:RCo 200 IU/dL or FVIII 250–300 IU/dL. Notably, 22 of the 41 subjects enrolled in the phase IV study of Humate-P with PK analysis were observed to have high levels of VWF:RCo and/or FVIII activity (range 1–8 days VWF:RCo, 2–7 days FVIII activity), and despite this, none developed thromboembolic disease (Di Paola et al., 2011).

Lastly, consideration for use of other therapies could be made. Antifibrinolytic therapy is commonly used as adjunct therapy for procedures involving the mucosa (oral cavity, gastrointestinal, and genitourinary tracts). Topical agents (topical thrombin, fibrin sealant) could be used in the surgical setting for minor bleeding or for wound bleeding. Though these are routinely used, and would be considered possibly useful adjunct agents in this clinical scenario, it should be noted that the safety of these agents has not been systematically investigated in vWD.

References

Di Paola J, Lethagen S, Gill J, *et al.* (2011) Presurgical pharmacokinetic analysis of a von Willebrand factor/factor VIII (VWF/FVIII) concentrate in patients with von Willebrand's disease (VWD) has limited value in dosing for surgery. *Haemophilia* **17**(5): 752–758.

Gill JC, Shapiro A, Valentino LA, *et al.* (2011) von Willebrand factor/factor VIII concentrate (Humate-P) for management of elective surgery in adults and children with von Willebrand disease. *Haemophilia* **17**(6): 895–905.

Humate-P [package insert], Marburg, Germany, CSL Berhring GmbH, 2010.

Nichols WL, *et al.* (2008) von Willebrand disease (VWD): evidence-based diagnosis and management guidelines. The National Heart, Lung, and Blood Institute (NHLBI) Expert Panel report (USA). *Haemophilia* **14**(2): 171–232.

Gynecologic and Obstetric Considerations:
von Willebrand Disease and Obstetric/Gynecologic Procedures

Alice D. Ma
Division of Hematology/Oncology, University of North Carolina, Chapel Hill, NC, USA

Recently, a number of our female patients with type 1 VWD, all of whom respond well to DDAVP, have been requiring GYN procedures. We thought it useful to codify our recommendations for management. Again, these recommendations are for women with type 1 VWD who have a good response to DDAVP.

1 For minor procedures such as insertion of a Mirena® IUD, we recommend pre-treatment with DDAVP, either IV or intranasally (Stimate®) 30–60 min prior to the procedure. An additional dose of Stimate ®may be required 1–2 days later.

2 For a cone biopsy or LEEP procedure or endometrial ablation, we typically recommend DDAVP, either IV or intranasally (Stimate®) 30–60 min prior to the procedure. Further Stimate® dosing should be given on post-operative days (PODs) 1 and 2. We recommend the use of epsilon amino-caproic acid, 50 mg/kg po q6 h × 1 week.

3 For any laparoscopic procedure, or for hysterectomy, we recommend the use of Humate-P, 40–60 RCo units/kg IV 30–60 min prior to the procedure. We recommend that this be given q 12 h for a total of three doses, then q 24 h to complete 3–5 days. We then recommend the use of Stimate nasal spray on POD s 7–9.

Hemophilia and Hemostasis: A Case-Based Approach to Management, Second Edition.
Edited by Alice D. Ma, Harold R. Roberts, Miguel A. Escobar.
© 2013 John Wiley & Sons, Ltd. Published 2013 by John Wiley & Sons, Ltd.

4 For pregnancy, it is important that obstetrics, anesthesia, pediatrics, and hematology are all involved with the birthing plan. We recommend against use of vacuum extraction and forceps. We do not recommend the routine use of Caesarean section, which should be performed for obstetrical indications only. Epidural and spinal anesthesia are contraindicated if there is a coagulation defect. There is no contraindication to regional anesthesia if coagulation is normalized, but the anesthesia service has final discretion over performing these procedures and may have a different assessment of bleeding risk. We try to follow VWF levels in the last trimester. If coagulation numbers have normalized, the patient should be at no increased risk of abnormal bleeding for vaginal delivery, Caesarean delivery, or regional anesthesia. Some patients fail to completely normalize their VWF levels, and these patients may require infusions of Humate-P prior to invasive procedures. The risk of early and late postpartum hemorrhage is increased in women with bleeding disorders. Women with inherited bleeding disorders should be advised about the possibility of excessive postpartum bleeding and instructed to report this immediately. Additionally, intramuscular injections, surgery, and circumcision should be avoided in neonates at risk for a severe hereditary bleeding disorder until adequate work-up/preparation are possible.

Reference

Demers C, Derzko C, David M, Douglas J; Society of Obstetricians and Gynecologists of Canada (2005) Gynaecological and obstetric management of women with inherited bleeding disorders. *J Obstet Gynaecol Can* **27**(7): 707–732.

Rare Forms of von Willebrand Disease

Type 2A von Willebrand Disease and Recurrent Gastrointestinal Bleeding

Alice D. Ma

Division of Hematology/Oncology, University of North Carolina, Chapel Hill, NC, USA

A 57-year-old man presented with a history of type 2A VWD and multiple GI bleeds. He was initially diagnosed with 2A VWD after having epistaxis and bleeding after tooth extractions. He initially had a GI bleed at age 50 (September 1995) and was found to have a hemoglobin value of 2.7 g/dL, an antral ulcer and duodenal AVM. One year later, he had gastric and esophageal ulcers. In November 1996, he was found to have AVMs in his small bowel and was started on estrogens, which he took for less than 2 years. In December of 1998, he was treated with Humate-P® for an episode of hematochezia. He was again given Humate-P® for hematochezia in September 2000 for presumed diverticular bleed. In January 2001, he was again tried on two other estrogen preparations for hematochezia. He began receiving more frequent doses of VWF-containing FVIII preparations, but continued to have frequent hematochezia. By December of 2001, he had recurrent hematochezia, despite being treated with desmopressin and Koate®. The bleeding would recur 2–3 days after Koate® infusions. By April 2003, he had bleeding, despite daily Koate® infusions and oral desmopressin. The patient was initially seen at our center in April 2004. He complained that his stools were bloody about 50% of the time. He estimated that he had undergone endoscopy at least 12 times over the previous 12 years. He had received in excess of 200 units of red cells, and had been found to have AVMs on at least half of the endoscopies.

The patient was again seen at our center in 2007, at which time a problem with frequent line infections was noted. He had five ports removed. In June of 2007, another line was removed and the patient was treated with antibiotics. In terms of GI bleeding, he had undergone

Hemophilia and Hemostasis: A Case-Based Approach to Management, Second Edition.
Edited by Alice D. Ma, Harold R. Roberts, Miguel A. Escobar.
© 2013 John Wiley & Sons, Ltd. Published 2013 by John Wiley & Sons, Ltd.

endoscopy seven times in 3 years. AVMs were invariably seen, but not cauterized. He had been treated with Humate-P®, given twice daily. He would receive IV iron at his internist's office.

Q	What alternative therapies could be tried at this time?

The patient was started on treatment with thalidomide, 50 mg daily. The dose was increased to 100 mg daily, but because of bloating and fatigue, the dose was decreased back to 50 mg daily and eventually discontinued in November 2008. Several case reports and case series have reported improvement in symptoms of chronic bleeding from AVMs with use of thalidomide, but patients may not be able to tolerate the drug due to side effects, as was the case in our patient.

The patient was noted to have a new heart murmur in 2008, and echocardiography done in December 2008 showed a 0.5-cm vegetation on the aortic valve and a 1.5-cm vegetation on the mitral valve. He underwent repair of his mitral valve and aortic valve replacement with a tissue valve. A PICC line was placed for antibiotic and factor administration. Notably, he had had an episode of endocarditis 7–8 years prior; 3 months previously, vegetations had been noted at an outside hospital and the patient had been treated with antibiotics. It was suspected that the patient had developed some degree of Heyde's syndrome, which is the concordance of acquired 2A VWD associated with high shear cardiac lesions and gastrointestinal AVMs. He remained on Humate-P® given thrice weekly for long term prophylaxis and had not had GI bleeding for over 16 months follow-up.

References

Hirri HM, Green PJ, Lindsay J (2006) Von Willebrand disease and angiodysplasia treated with thalidomide. *Haemophilia* **12**: 285–286.

Kamalaporn P, Saravanan R, Cirocco M, *et al.* (2009) Thalidomide for the treatment of chronic gastrointestinal bleeding from angiodysplasias: a case series. *Eur J Gastroenterol Hepatol* **21**: 1347–1350.

Makris M (2006) Gastrointestinal bleeding in von Willebrand disease. *Thromb Res* **118S**(1): S13–17.

Nomikou E, Tsevrenis V, Gafou A, *et al.* (2009) Type IIb von Willebrand disease with angiodysplasias and refractory gastrointestinal bleeding successfully treated with thalidomide. *Haemophilia* **15**:1340–1342.

CASE STUDY 32

Type 2B von Willebrand Disease and Thoracic Surgery

Alice D. Ma

Division of Hematology/Oncology, University of North Carolina, Chapel Hill, NC, USA

A 75-year-old man with a history of type 2B VWD presented with a spiculated lung mass suspicious for lung cancer. He is scheduled for thoracic surgery – likely to include left upper lobectomy. He was initially diagnosed in his 50s after his daughter was diagnosed after suffering severe hemorrhage following a stillbirth. He has had lifelong nosebleeds and recurrent iron deficiency anemia, felt to be due to GI bleeding from a number of sources, including gastric polyps, hemorrhoids, and small bowel AVMs. His baseline platelet count runs between 25 and 60×10^9/L.

Q	How should he be managed around the time of his surgery?

Type 2B von Willebrand disease is frequently associated with thrombocytopenia due to accelerated clearance of the platelets along with the high molecular weight multimers of VWD, which exhibit enhanced adhesion to the platelets. For this reason, in addition to replacing VWF with a VWF-containing FVIII concentrate, platelets frequently need to be transfused as well, especially during major surgical procedures. DDAVP should not be used for major surgery. We recommended that the patient receive 60 RCo units/kg of Humate-P® immediately pre-operatively and every 8 h for 2 days, then q12 × 7 days. We recommended a transfusion of platelets immediately pre-operatively and platelet count checks to keep the platelet count between 80 and 100×10^9/dL.

Hemophilia and Hemostasis: A Case-Based Approach to Management, Second Edition.
Edited by Alice D. Ma, Harold R. Roberts, Miguel A. Escobar.
© 2013 John Wiley & Sons, Ltd. Published 2013 by John Wiley & Sons, Ltd.

CASE STUDY 33

von Willebrand Disease 2N

Tzu-Fei Wang[1] and Alice D. Ma[2]

[1] Divisions of Hematology and Oncology, Washington University School of Medicine, Saint Louis, MO, USA

[2] Division of Hematology/Oncology, University of North Carolina, Chapel Hill, NC, USA

A 30-year-old female presented with a life-long history of abnormal bleeding from the nose, gums, and teeth, and heavy menstrual bleeding. In high school, she had a left lower extremity hematoma associated with a sports injury, requiring surgical intervention. Due to these abnormal episodes, an evaluation for a bleeding diathesis was undertaken. She was found to have normal levels of von Willebrand factor (VWF) antigen and activity on multiple occasions; however, the factor VIII level was found to be low at 16–22% repeatedly. A platelet function test (PFA-100®) was normal, and her aPTT was about 1.4 times of upper limit of normal. Her paternal grandmother and sister carried no formal diagnoses, but were reported to have significant bruising. A DDAVP trial showed a satisfactory response, with factor VIII level rising 5 times compared to her baseline (23% to 121% at 1 h). Therefore, DDAVP was used pre-operatively for an elective right-hand surgery. However, 3 days after the operation, she developed significant swelling and bruising consistent with delayed hemorrhage at the surgical site. Hemostasis was subsequently achieved with infusions of VWF-containing FVIII concentrate. A genetic analysis showed homozygous mutation from arginine to glutamine at codon 854 in exon 20 of the VWF gene, confirming the diagnosis of von Willebrand Normandy (VWD type 2N) disease.

Q1	How does this disorder differ from other forms of von Willebrand disease?

von Willebrand type 2N disease is a rare autosomal recessive bleeding disorder. The prevalence is estimated to be 1–5 per million population,

Hemophilia and Hemostasis: A Case-Based Approach to Management, Second Edition.
Edited by Alice D. Ma, Harold R. Roberts, Miguel A. Escobar.
© 2013 John Wiley & Sons, Ltd. Published 2013 by John Wiley & Sons, Ltd.

accounting for 1–2% of all VWD and 13% of all type 2 VWD (Favaloro *et al.*, 2009). "N" stands for Normandy in France, where the first patient was described in 1990 (Mazurier *et al.*, 1990). Many mis-sense mutations have been identified in the N terminal of VWF, the binding site of factor VIII, resulting in its defective binding to factor VIII. Without binding to and being protected by VWF, circulating factor VIII is susceptible to proteolysis, resulting in decreased levels of factor VIII, generally to 5–15% of normal. As a result, patients can present with symptoms similar to those of mild hemophilia A, such as joint or muscle bleeding, rather than mucocutaneous bleeding which is generally seen in other types of VWD. VWF antigen and activity levels are normal in classic type 2N VWD. However, individuals may be compound heterozygotes for type 1 VWD and 2N VWD, in which case the FVIII levels will be lower than expected in a typical type 1 patient.

Q2	How does one differentiate a von Willebrand Normandy patient from a symptomatic carrier of hemophilia A?

VWD 2N should be considered in females with bleeding symptoms resembling hemophilia A, or patients with a family history of autosomal inheritance pattern. The classic laboratory findings include normal VWF antigen and activity, with disproportionally low factor VIII level. These patients are easily misdiagnosed as symptomatic carriers of hemophilia A or other types of VWD. The latter happens when a patient has compound heterozygous mutation, resulting in decreased VWF activity and/or antigen levels. To differentiate VWD 2N from a symptomatic carrier state of hemophilia A, VWF–FVIII binding (VWF:FVIIIB) assay or genetic analysis to detect mutations in VWF and/or factor VIII are needed.

Q3	How should her management be improved for future surgeries to ensure adequate hemostasis?

Desmopressin (DDAVP) trials are routinely obtained in patients with VWD or mild hemophilia A. Increase in factor levels indicates response to DDAVP and potential use for hemostasis in the setting of injury, trauma, or bleeding. DDAVP alone should not be used in VWD 2N, especially in the setting of a major surgery. The released factor VIII remains susceptible to proteolysis and suffers from a short half-life due to its poor binding to VWF. To confirm the presence of the accelerated clearance of factor VIII, a factor VIII level should be measured at 4 h post-DDAVP, in addition to the standard 1 h post-DDAVP. An increased clearance of factor VIII was the most likely etiology of delayed hemorrhage in our patient. Therefore, VWF concentrate infusion is the treatment of choice in patients with VWD 2N with major bleeding, surgery, or trauma. Factor VIII concentrates without VWF (e.g. recombinant FVIII) should not be used for this disease.

References

Favaloro EJ, Mohammed S, Koutts J (2009) Identification and prevalence of von Willebrand disease type 2N (Normandy) in Australia. *Blood Coag Fibrin* **20**: 706–714.

Mazurier C, Dieval J, Jorieux S, *et al.* (1990) A new von Willebrand factor (vWF) defect in a patient with factor VIII (FVIII) deficiency but with normal levels and multimeric patterns of both plasma and platelet vWF. Characterization of abnormal vWF/FVIII interaction. *Blood* **75**: 20–26.

Peerlinck K, Eikenboom K, Ploos Van Amstel HK, *et al.* (1992) A patient with von Willebrand's disease characterized by a compound heterozygosity for a substitution of Arg 854 by Gln in the putative factor-VIII-binding domain of von Willebrand factor (vWF) on one allele and very low levels of mRNA from the second vWF allele. *Br J Haematol* **80**: 358–363.

PART III
Other Bleeding Disorders

CASE STUDY 34

Prothrombin Deficiency

Alice D. Ma

Division of Hematology/Oncology, University of North Carolina, Chapel Hill, NC, USA

A 42-year-old woman with a lifelong history of mucocutaneous and post- surgical bleeding presented for evaluation. The patient's bleeding history is as follows. The patient has always complained of significant menorrhagia. In fact with her first menstrual cycle, she bled to a hemoglobin of 6.5 g/dL. When she is not on oral contraceptive pills, her menses last between 7 and 14 days, requiring changing a pad or tampon two or three times per hour. She has required transfusions on a number of occasions. She has required exploratory laparotomies and D&Cs.

The patient underwent rhinoplasty in Canada in her 20s. Her surgery was complicated by significant excessive bleeding and she was seen by a hematologist in Canada who told her she had a low factor II level.

At age 25, the patient underwent wisdom tooth extraction and had no excessive bleeding, though she was treated with topical liquid epsilon amino-caproic acid. She recently moved to South Carolina and had an episode of heavy menstrual bleeding requiring blood transfusion, exploratory laparotomy and D&C. She married in 2007 and because of hopes for fertility, was seen at our center. Family history is notable for parents who are first cousins.

Here, she had a factor II activity level of 15%, with all other factor levels within normal limits. The PFA-100® was also within normal limits. The PT was slightly prolonged at 15.8 sec and corrected with 1:1 mix. The factor II level was repeated and was again found to be low at 14%.

Q1	How should she be treated for menorrhagia, given her desire for fertility?

Hemophilia and Hemostasis: A Case-Based Approach to Management, Second Edition.
Edited by Alice D. Ma, Harold R. Roberts, Miguel A. Escobar.
© 2013 John Wiley & Sons, Ltd. Published 2013 by John Wiley & Sons, Ltd.

The patient was placed on epsiolon aminocaproic acid, which she takes between 1 g and 3 g daily during her menses. She notes that when she takes 3 g daily her menses cease. She normally takes approximately 1–2 g daily during her menstrual cycle and notes significant improvement in menorrhagia.

Q2	The patient eventually underwent IVF with donor eggs. How should she be treated for her delivery?

Factor II is found in Prothrombin complex concentrates (PCCs). PCCs currently available in the United States include Bebulin VH® (Baxter) and Profilnine SD® (Grifols). These products vary in their factor content, with Bebulin showing X>II>IX>VII and Profilnine having II>IX=X>VII. Both are virally inactivated plasma-derived products. In her third trimester, she had no change in her baseline FII activity level. Our recommendations were to treat the patient with Profilnine at a dose of 30–50 units/kg, keeping FII levels between 20 and 40%. Unfortunately, she chose to deliver at a center that had no capacity to measure FII levels. It is not clear whether she had PT/PTT monitoring. She delivered by Caesarean section and lost in excess of 2L of blood.

References

http://www.hemophilia.org/NHFWeb/MainPgs/MainNHF.aspx?menuid=57& contentid=693. These are the MASAC recommendations concerning products licensed for the treatment of hemophilia and other bleeding disorders *(revised May 2011)*.
http://www.hemophilia.org/NHFWeb/Resource/StaticPages/menu0/menu5/menu57/masac190tables.pdf. Table V gives the relative concentrations of the PCCs.

CASE STUDY 35

Factor V Deficiency

Miguel A. Escobar

Division of Hematology, University of Texas Health Science Center at Houston and Gulf States Hemophilia and Thrombophilia Center, Houston, TX, USA

A 51-year-old Caucasian female was brought by the EMS with mental changes and headache. Screening coagulation studies showed a prolonged PT: 41.8 sec (normal 8.8–11.3 sec) and PTT: 147 sec (normal 24–35.6 sec). She also had a mild microcytic anemia from iron deficiency. A 1:1 mixing study showed complete correction of the PT and PTT. Further evaluation showed a large subdural hematoma without evidence of fracture and a factor V activity of <1%. She was treated with fresh frozen plasma every 24 h for 7 days. Once neurologically recovered she was able to relate a history of factor V deficiency and chronic menorrhagia and epistaxis. She has taken iron supplements intermittently for many years. Surprisingly, she had no previous life-threatening hemorrhages. She had suffered a single traumatic knee hemarthrosis.

Congenital factor V deficiency is a rare (1:1 million) autosomal recessive disorder. Factor V is found in the plasma and the alpha granules of platelets. About 20% of the total body pool of factor V is stored in the platelets. Clinical manifestations can be mild, moderate, or severe. Some patients with factor V levels below 1% have minimal bleeding complications, suggesting that platelet factor V plays an important role in hemostasis. Laboratory evaluation reveals a prolonged PT and PTT with a normal thrombin time. Definite diagnosis requires a factor V assay.

A differential diagnosis must consider an acquired factor V deficiency from liver disease, DIC, and inhibitors against factor V which, although rare, can sometimes occur during exposure to antibiotics or infections. Some patients develop antibodies to factor V when they are exposed to

Hemophilia and Hemostasis: A Case-Based Approach to Management, Second Edition.
Edited by Alice D. Ma, Harold R. Roberts, Miguel A. Escobar.
© 2013 John Wiley & Sons, Ltd. Published 2013 by John Wiley & Sons, Ltd.

topical bovine thrombin that contains bovine factor V which cross-reacts with human factor V.

The treatment of choice for moderate to severe bleeds is fresh frozen plasma since there are no commercially-available factor V concentrates. For minor bleeds, local measures and antifibrinolytics can be used. With the use of plasma the goal is to achieve levels close to 25% of normal. Plasma can be given as an initial loading dose of 15–20 mL/kg of body weight, followed by 3–6 mL/kg of body weight every 24h given the long half-life of factor V (~36h). Recombinant FVIIa has been reported to stop bleeding in some patients with factor V deficiency.

Reference

Roberts HR, Escobar MA (2007) Less common congenital disorders of hemostasis. In: Kitchens CS, *et al.* (eds.), *Consultative Hemostasis and Thrombosis* (2nd edn.). W.B. Saunders Company.

CASE STUDY 36

Factor VII Deficiency

Trinh T. Nguyen and Miguel A. Escobar

Division of Hematology, University of Texas Health Science Center at Houston and Gulf States Hemophilia and Thrombophilia Center, Houston, TX, USA

A 35-year-old Asian woman with mild factor VII deficiency, baseline level 49%, presented for pre-operative evaluation prior to parathyroidectomy. She had no other bleeding symptoms aside from menometrorrhagia.

Q1	What is the appropriate management for this patient when she undergoes surgery?

Bleeding in patients with factor VII deficiency does not necessarily correlate with factor levels. Factor VII levels <10% are typically associated with a more severe bleeding diathesis, but even patients with levels <1% do not always have severe bleeding. This patient has a FVII level well above the recommended threshold for surgery, which is a goal of >15% pre-operatively. Aside from menorrhagia, she had no other bleeding manifestations. As such, we did not recommend prophylactic factor VII replacement prior to surgical resection of her parathyroid.

She developed leg pain and swelling 7 days post-operatively. Imaging was consistent with deep vein thrombosis of the right common femoral vein.

Q2	What is the appropriate management of this patient now?

Similar to factor XII deficiency and dysfibrinogenemias, factor VII deficiency does not offer protection against thromboembolic events. Mariani *et al.* (2003) could not identify phenotypic and molecular-genetic markers to

Hemophilia and Hemostasis: A Case-Based Approach to Management, Second Edition.
Edited by Alice D. Ma, Harold R. Roberts, Miguel A. Escobar.
© 2013 John Wiley & Sons, Ltd. Published 2013 by John Wiley & Sons, Ltd.

identify those at higher risk of thrombosis in their evaluation of patients from the FVII Deficiency Study Group database. Patients with factor deficiencies who develop thrombosis require anticoagulation, as does any patient without a bleeding disorder. This patient was started on full dose enoxaparin and bridged to Coumadin with goal INR 2-3. She completed 6 months of therapy with resolution of thrombus and no bleeding complications

References

Barnett JM (2005) Lack of bleeding in patients with severe factor VII deficiency. *Am J Hematol* **78**(2): 134–137.

Giansily-Blaizot M (2004) Analysis of biological phenotypes from 42 patients with inherited factor VII deficiency: can biological tests predict the bleeding risk? *Haemotologica* **89**(6): 704–709.

Mariani G, *et al.* (2003) Thrombosis in inherited factor VII deficiency. *J Thromb Haemost* **1**(10): 2153–2158.

Roberts HR, Escobar MA (2007) Less common congenital disorders of hemostasis. In: Kitchens CS *et al.* (eds.), *Consultative Hemostasis and Thrombosis* (2nd edn.). Philadelphia, PA: Saunders Elsevier, pp. 61–79.

Factor X Deficiency

Alice D. Ma

Division of Hematology/Oncology, University of North Carolina, Chapel Hill, NC, USA

A 47-year-old woman with a history of FX deficiency, baseline level 3–7% presented for evaluation. She was initially diagnosed at our center in 1987. Her mother had been noted to have FX of 57%. At age 17, the patient had bleeding for 3 months following a sports injury. She has had lifelong epistaxis and menorrhagia.

She had wisdom teeth removed w/FFP in 1986, had tonsillectomy with Proplex×2 doses and SD-FFP in 1999, had trigger thumb repaired with solvent-detergent-treated fresh frozen plasma (SD-FFP).

Currently, the patient has multiple broken teeth. She underwent local anesthesia, after which "her face blew up." The patient went to the ER, was given 3 units FFP, developed hives, and wheezing.

Q1. How should this patient be treated for her upcoming dental surgery?

FX is found in Prothrombin complex concentrates (PCCs). PCCs currently available in the United States include Bebulin VH (Baxter) and Profilnine SD (Grifols). These products both vary in their factor content, with Bebulin showing X>II>IX>VII and Profilnine having II>IX=X>VII, and b oth are virally inactivated plasma-derived products. We recommend the use of Profilnine at a dose of 30 units/kg immediately prior to tooth extractions. The patient should be pre-medicated with diphenhydramine prior to factor administration. We also recommend the use of a 25% solution of epsilon aminocaproic acid at a dose of 50 mg/kg given swish and swallow every 6 h for 7–10 days.

Hemophilia and Hemostasis: A Case-Based Approach to Management, Second Edition.
Edited by Alice D. Ma, Harold R. Roberts, Miguel A. Escobar.
© 2013 John Wiley & Sons, Ltd. Published 2013 by John Wiley & Sons, Ltd.

References

http://www.hemophilia.org/NHFWeb/MainPgs/MainNHF.aspx?menuid=57&
  contentid=693. These are the MASAC recommendations concerning products licensed
  for the treatment of hemophilia and other bleeding disorders (revised May 2011).
http://www.hemophilia.org/NHFWeb/Resource/StaticPages/menu0/menu5/menu57/
  masac190tables.pdf. Table V gives the relative concentrations of the PCCs.

CASE STUDY 38

Factor XI Deficiency

Trinh T. Nguyen and Miguel A. Escobar

Division of Hematology, University of Texas Health Science Center at Houston and Gulf States Hemophilia and Thrombophilia Center, Houston, TX, USA

A 15-year-old Hispanic teenager presented to the hematology clinic with a microcytic hypochromic anemia and menorrhagia. Menses were noted over the last 7–9 days, with significant flow the first several days and occasional overflowing. Work up by her PCP included an elevated PTT of 45 sec. The patient also complained of easy bruising and occasional epistaxis. There is a family history of easy bruising, epistaxis, and menorrhagia in her mother and older sister. Neither have been formally diagnosed with a bleeding disorder. Her brothers also have frequent epistaxis but otherwise no bleeding diathesis.

Q1	What is the diagnostic work up for this patient?

Iron deficiency anemia is common in menstruating females. However, with the history of excessive menstrual bleeding in her mother and sister, as well as epistaxis in her brothers, one must wonder if there is an underlying bleeding disorder in this family. Her PTT is elevated, suggesting factor deficiency, and the diagnostic evaluation of such a patient includes factors VIII, IX, XI, XII, and von Willebrand studies. Liver function should also be tested as most coagulation factors are made by the liver. For this patient, work up revealed normal von Willebrand factor and ristocetin activity and normal coagulation factors except for a low factor XI of 22%.

Q2	What therapeutic options are available for her menorrhagia?

Hemophilia and Hemostasis: A Case-Based Approach to Management, Second Edition.
Edited by Alice D. Ma, Harold R. Roberts, Miguel A. Escobar.
© 2013 John Wiley & Sons, Ltd. Published 2013 by John Wiley & Sons, Ltd.

Unlike hemophilia A and B, hemophilia C (aka Rosenthal syndrome, factor XI deficiency) is transmitted via an autosomal inheritance pattern. Severely affected patients have levels <15%. Heterozygotes have levels 20–70% of normal. Similar to factor VII deficiency, the severity of bleeding does not correspond to factor XI levels. Also unlike hemophilia A and B, hemophilia C is not typically associated with spontaneous muscle or joint bleedings. Rather, patients with this disorder typically present with easy bruising, epistaxis, and/or bleeding following surgery or trauma. In fact, most patients are asymptomatic until hemostatically challenged. Even within surgical challenges, bleeding manifestations are variable depending on the site of surgery. Areas with high fibrinolytic activity – nasal or oral cavity, prostate – tend to bleed more readily than elsewhere. In girls, menorrhagia is a common presenting symptom and factor XI deficiency must be considered in the differential diagnosis of such patients.

Q3	Should she receive prophylaxis if she undergoes surgery?

In the US, there is no readily available factor XI concentrate. Bleeding in factor XI patients are treated with antifibrinolytics – aminocaproic acid or tranexemic acid. FFP may be used if breakthrough bleeding occurs with antifibrinolytics. Recombinant factor VIIa is another option for refractory bleeding although optimal dosing has not been established. Topical agents such as thrombin and fibrin glue are also options for post-operative nasal or oral cavity surgeries. For menstruating females, oral contraceptive pills can help to regulate menorrhagia as well as limit blood loss and subsequent iron deficiency anemia; however, antifibrinolytics are usually adequate to prevent significant blood loss in these patients.

References

Gomez K (2008) Factor XI deficiency. *Haemophilia* **14**: 1183–1189.

O'Connell NM (2004) Factor XI deficiency. *Semin Hematol* **41**(Suppl 1): 76–81.

Salomon O, Steinberg DM, Seligshon U (2006) Variable bleeding manifestations characterize different types of surgery in patients with severe factor XI deficiency enabling parsimonious use of replacement therapy. *Haemophilia* **12**: 490–493.

CASE STUDY 39

Factor XIII Deficiency

Alice D. Ma

Division of Hematology/Oncology, University of North Carolina, Chapel Hill, NC, USA

A 5-year-old boy presented for the evaluation of abnormal bleeding. He was the product of an uncomplicated delivery to a 24-year-old Guatemalan woman. 7 lb 4 oz boy, underwent circumcision without difficulty. During days 1–7 of life, he had umbilical stump bleeding, showing a "ring of blood" on his T-shirt. On Day 8 the umbilical stump fell off, leading to profound bleeding. Despite suturing, the patient continued to have bleeding enough to saturate bandages. Family history was notable for a maternal great uncle with poor wound healing and death due to intracranial hemorrhage as a teenager. At our center, clot lysis time was <2 h, consistent with FXIII deficiency.

Q	How should the patient be treated?

Patients with FXIII deficiency are at very high risk (30%) for spontaneous intracranial hemorrhage, and it is therefore recommended that all patients, even asymptomatic patients, receive prophylaxis with FXIII concentrates, which are now available. Fibrogammin P® is a purified, pasteurized concentrate of FXIII that appears to carry negligible risk of viral transmission, unlike other unprocessed products containing FXIII, such as FFP and cryoprecipitate. Due to its long half-life (7–12 days), Fibrogammin® P can be administered for prophylactic treatment once every 3–4 weeks. Scheduled monthly treatment with 10–30 units/kg of Fibrogammin® P is considered sufficient in most cases to maintain FXIII levels above a critical threshold to prevent bleeding episodes.

Hemophilia and Hemostasis: A Case-Based Approach to Management, Second Edition.
Edited by Alice D. Ma, Harold R. Roberts, Miguel A. Escobar.
© 2013 John Wiley & Sons, Ltd. Published 2013 by John Wiley & Sons, Ltd.

References

Muszbek L, Bagoly Z, Cairo A, Peyvandi F (2011) Novel aspects of factor XIII deficiency. *Curr Opin Hematol* **18**: 366–372.

Lusher J, Pipe SW, Alexander S, Nugent D (2010) Prophylactic therapy with Fibrogammin P is associated with a decreased incidence of bleeding episodes: a retrospective study. *Haemophilia*. **16**: 316–321.

CASE STUDY 40

Combined Factor V and Factor VIII Deficiency

Tyler Buckner and Alice D. Ma

Division of Hematology/Oncology, University of North Carolina, Chapel Hill, NC, USA

My patient and his brother have combined factor V and factor VIII deficiency (Zhang et al., 2003; Spreafico and Peyvandi, 2008). His baseline FVIII level is 12%. His FV level is 10%. He has had abnormal bleeding with prior surgical procedures.

Q1	How is this condition different from other bleeding disorders?

Combined factor V and factor VIII deficiency (F5F8D) is a rare autosomal recessive bleeding disorder, with an estimated incidence of about 1 in 1 million in the general population. The incidence is increased to as high as 1 in 100,000 in the Middle Eastern Jewish and Iranian populations. F5F8D affects men and women in equal numbers, and patients with F5F8D account for about 3% of the rare bleeding disorder population world wide.

F5F8D is caused by a deficiency in intracellular transport of the (normal) factor V and factor VIII proteins from the endoplasmic reticulum to the Golgi apparatus. The underlying defects identified at the time of this writing are found in one of two proteins: either the ER-to-Golgi transport protein LMAN1 (lectin mannose binding protein) or MCFD2 (multiple coagulation factor deficiency 2), which is a cofactor for LMAN1.

Patients with F5F8D have mild to moderate bleeding symptoms, characterized by easy bruising, epistaxis, gum bleeding, bleeding with surgery and dental extractions, menorrhagia, and post-partum hemorrhage. Hemarthroses and soft tissue hematomas are unusual. Both the PT

Hemophilia and Hemostasis: A Case-Based Approach to Management, Second Edition.
Edited by Alice D. Ma, Harold R. Roberts, Miguel A. Escobar.
© 2013 John Wiley & Sons, Ltd. Published 2013 by John Wiley & Sons, Ltd.

and aPTT are prolonged, and platelet count and function are normal. Factor V and factor VIII activity levels are usually in the 5–20% range.

Patients with newly diagnosed mild deficiency of FVIII without a family history of hemophilia A should have FV levels measured to rule out this rare disorder.

Q2	How should I manage his coagulopathy during an elective rotator cuff repair?

Treatment of bleeding or prevention of intra- and post-operative bleeding in patients with F5F8D is accomplished primarily by infusion of exogenous factor V and factor VIII.

Factor VIII can be replaced using either recombinant or plasma-derived factor VIII concentrates. Desmopressin (DDAVP) may be used in patients who show an appropriate rise in factor VIII levels after a test dose of DDAVP. The goal for FVIII levels is the same as in other patients with FVIII deficiency.

Factor V is replaced with plasma infusions, but the volume required may be limiting. Our patient had previously been treated with 30 mL FFP/kg prior to a cardiac catheterization procedure, but developed pulmonary edema and a non-ST-elevation myocardial infarction.

Plasma exchange is an alternative means of increasing factor V levels in cases in which the volume of FFP is a limiting factor. Remember that ACE inhibitors should be stopped prior to plasma exchange procedures. Our patient developed hypotension and dyspnea during his plasma exchange procedure done prior to his coronary artery bypass procedure. He had been on enalapril which had not been discontinued appropriately. In cases where plasma exchange or plasma infusions cannot be used, platelet transfusion may be used, since 20% of the body's factor V resides in platelets. This patient has subsequently been treated with platelet transfusions along with his FVIII replacement without difficulty or hemorrhage prior to many other surgical procedures.

Antifibrinolytic medications (such as epsilon aminocaproic acid or tranexamic acid) are sometimes useful adjunctive treatments for minor mucosal bleeding.

Goal levels for each factor vary by the clinical severity of the bleeding and/or the planned operative procedure. Target levels for minor bleeds and surgical procedures are at least 15 IU/dL for factor V and 30–50 IU/dL for factor VIII. Major bleeding and surgical procedures require levels of at least 20–25 IU/dL for factor V and 50–70 IU/dL for factor VIII.

References

Spreafico M, Peyvandi F (2008) Combined FV and FVIII deficiency. *Haemophilia* **14**(6): 1201–1208.

Zhang B, Cunningham MA, Nichols WC, *et al.* (2003) Bleeding due to disruption of a cargo-specific ER-to-Golgi transport complex. *Nature Genet* **34**(2): 220–225.

CASE STUDY 41

Glanzmann Thrombaesthenia

Alice D. Ma

Division of Hematology/Oncology, University of North Carolina, Chapel Hill, NC, USA

A 26-year-old Hispanic man, stabbed 8 times in anterior chest/abdomen, arrived at our center via ambulance. He was hypotensive and short of breath. BP 67/38, HR 130's, RR 30's. He was only able to say "Hemofilia." CXR showed bilateral pneumothoraces. The patient was taken emergently to the OR after intubation and placement of bilateral chest tubes. The right-sided chest tube drained 750 cc blood. Blood products were empirically given, including PRBCs, platelets, FFP, and cryoprecipitate. In the OR, the patient was noted to have two large liver lacerations, which were treated with laser photocoagulation. Cardiothoracic surgery was called to evaluate profound drainage from the chest tube – a total of 1,900 cc of blood. Rather than perform thoracotomy, the surgeons opted to treat the patient with recombinant activated FVII. The patient subsequently had no further drainage from his chest tubes.

At this point, a hematology consultation was obtained. All coagulation screens were normal, and factor activity levels were normal or supranormal. However, 5 days post-operatively, all wounds began to ooze. The patient developed epistaxis and UGI bleeding. PT and aPTT were normal. The PFA-100 ® showed infinite closure times in both the collagen/epinephrine and collagen/ADP cartridges. The patient was given DDAVP and a platelet transfusion with resolution of bleeding.

Q1	How should the patient be evaluated further?

Hemophilia and Hemostasis: A Case-Based Approach to Management, Second Edition.
Edited by Alice D. Ma, Harold R. Roberts, Miguel A. Escobar.
© 2013 John Wiley & Sons, Ltd. Published 2013 by John Wiley & Sons, Ltd.

The patient was followed up in clinic. With the assistance of a translator, a history of severe nosebleeds, requiring transfusions was obtained. The patient's brother (one of 8 siblings) also had severe nosebleeds and bruising. The PT and aPTT again were normal. PFA-100 ® again showed infinite closure times with col/epi and col/ADP cartridges. Platelet aggregation studies showed no response to thrombin, collagen, ADP, epinephrine, or arachidonic acid. Normal agglutination occurred in response to ristocetin. Platelet electron microscopy showed no binding of gold-labeled fibrinogen to the patient's platelets, confirming the diagnosis of Glanzmann's thrombasthenia.

Glanzmann thrombasthenia is a rare autosomal recessive disorder in which patients fail to express glycoprotein IIbIIIa on the platelet surface, leading to an absence of platelet aggregation. Patients have a severe bleeding phenotype, exhibiting mucocutaneous and post-surgical bleeding. Severe bleeding should be treated with platelet transfusions, but alloimmunization may limit the efficacy in later life. Recombinant activated FVII has been used successfully in this disorder and is approved in Europe for this indication.

References

Di Minno G, Coppola A, Di Minno MN, Poon MC (2009) Glanzmann's thrombasthenia (defective platelet integrin alphaIIb-beta3): proposals for management between evidence and open issues. *Thromb Haemost* **102**: 1157–1164.

Franchini M, Favaloro EJ, Lippi G (2010) Glanzmann thrombasthenia: an update. *Clin Chim Acta* **411**(1–2): 1–6.

CASE STUDY 42

Gardner–Diamond Syndrome and von Willebrand Disease

Tzu-Fei Wang[1] and Alice D. Ma[2]

[1] Divisions of Hematology and Oncology, Washington University School of Medicine, Saint Louis, MO, USA

[2] Division of Hematology/Oncology, University of North Carolina, Chapel Hill, NC, USA

A 31-year-old female presented with complaints of easy bruising for 6–12 months. She had a history of prolonged bleeding after wisdom teeth removal 11 years prior to presentation and a long history of heavy menstrual bleeding and endometriosis requiring multiple abdominal laparoscopic procedures and hysterectomy at the age of 25 years. She also had a breast biopsy resulting in a large hematoma requiring surgical evacuation. She reported bruises mostly appearing on her extremities. They were not related to trauma, appeared and disappeared synchronously in similar stages and colors, with central clearing, and were both palpable and painful. She noticed prodromal symptoms including joint pain and worsening fatigue prior to the onset of bruises. She had history of depression and anxiety, and significant stress with a recent divorce and was taking care of her children who also had health issues. She is not aware of a significant family history of bleeding disorders. Further work-up revealed a markedly abnormal PFA-100®. von Willebrand factor (VWF) antigen and activity levels were both at low normal range (40–45%). FVIII activity level was 60% of normal.

Q	What is her diagnosis, and what is the appropriate management?

Given her abnormal history of bleeding, abnormal PFA-100® and her VWF antigen and activity levels, which were lower than expected given significant stress, she was felt to have possible mild type 1 von Willebrand

Hemophilia and Hemostasis: A Case-Based Approach to Management, Second Edition.
Edited by Alice D. Ma, Harold R. Roberts, Miguel A. Escobar.
© 2013 John Wiley & Sons, Ltd. Published 2013 by John Wiley & Sons, Ltd.

disease (VWD). In addition, her symptoms of bruising were thought to be characteristic of Gardner–Diamond syndrome.

Gardner–Diamond syndrome, also called autoerythrocyte sensitization syndrome or psychogenic purpura, is a rare blood dyscrasia. It was first described in 1955 by Frank Gardner and Louis Diamond in four young females with a history of psychiatric disorders. The ecchymoses were characteristic for their synchronous appearance, morphology of central clearing, and frequent painful prodromes. The initial episode may be associated with trauma, but patients may then remit and relapse for many years spontaneously (Ivanov *et al.* 2009). Gardner and Diamond proposed that these patients developed sensitivity to extravasated red blood cells, since they all developed painful ecchymoses after intradermal injection of their own red blood cells. The optimal treatment for this disease is unclear. Therapies such as corticosteroids, contraceptives, and antibiotics have been tested in the past without significant efficacy (Ivanov *et al.* 2009). Hamblin *et al.* (1981) reported a case of autoerythrocyte sensitization to be effectively treated with plasmapheresis. Symptoms returned after plasmapheresis was replaced with sham procedures, refuting any potential placebo effect. Treatments for concurrent psychiatric disorders are also found to assist in symptom relief.

The laboratory hemostatic evaluation of Gardner–Diamond syndrome is typically normal (Gardner and Diamond 1955; Ivanov *et al.* 2009). Although this patient presented with abnormal PFA-100® and low normal VWF antigen and activity levels, her symptoms were so characteristic of Gardner–Diamond syndrome that we felt she may have two concurrent diagnoses, resulting in worse ecchymoses. Her PFA-100® normalized after desmopressin (DDAVP). Therefore, prophylactic nasal DDAVP was prescribed once weekly, aiming to improve her symptoms of painful ecchymoses. However, she developed painful migraines with visual symptoms after each dose of DDAVP. She is therefore undergoing a trial of plasmapheresis. She was encouraged to continue her psychological therapies as well.

References

Gardner FH, Diamond LK (1955) Autoerythrocyte sensitization. A form of purpura pro-ducing painful bruising following autosensitization to red blood cells in certain women. *Blood* **10**: 675–690.

Hamblin TJ, Hart S, Mufti GJ (1981) Plasmapheresis and a placebo procedure in auto-erythrocyte sensitization. *Br Med J* **283**: 1575–1576.

Ivanov OL, Lvov AN, Michenko AV, *et al.* (2009) Autoerythrocyte sensitization syndrome (Gardner–Diamond syndrome): review of the literature. *J Eur Acad Dermatol Venereol* **23**: 499–504.

CASE STUDY 43

Qualitative Platelet Disorder

Trinh T. Nguyen[1] and Miguel A. Escobar[2]
[1]Division of Hematology, University of Texas Health Science Center at Houston
[2]Gulf States Hemophilia and Thrombophilia Center, Houston, TX, USA

A 27-year-old Caucasian woman presented to the HTC for evaluation of QPD after her 2-year-old son was evaluated by the HTC for QPD. The son had presented with a 1.5 month history of nose bleeds. Family history was significant for the boy's mother having easy bruising, epistaxis, and menses lasting 7–9 days with overflowing and "doubling up" with both pads and tampons. After the son's labs were found to be concerning for qualitative platelet disorder, the patient was seen in clinic for evaluation. Her work-up was normal except for abnormal platelet aggregation – poor aggregation to arachidonic acid (both high and low doses), ADP low dose, collagen, epinephrine (H and L doses).

Q1	When should you consider work up of a patient with QPD?

Many women with menorrhagia do not realize they have a bleeding disorder. As such, the incidence of QPD and the more common von Willebrand disease are truly underestimated. Women with a bleeding disorder often come to the attention of the physician once their child is diagnosed with a bleeding disorder. This is the perfect case of the woman with a bleeding disorder not realizing she has any disorder at all.

Work-up of any bleeding disorder starts with a history and physical examination. Bleeding manifestations vary, depending on the underlying disorder. Spontaneous joint bleeding, for example, is rarely seen in QPD. Patients may present with easy bruising, epistaxis, and prolonged bleeding from surgical sites. The first line of work-up includes looking for the

Hemophilia and Hemostasis: A Case-Based Approach to Management, Second Edition.
Edited by Alice D. Ma, Harold R. Roberts, Miguel A. Escobar.
© 2013 John Wiley & Sons, Ltd. Published 2013 by John Wiley & Sons, Ltd.

more common causes of bleeding/bruising such as a CBC to rule out thrombocytopenia, PT/PTT and liver function assays for factor deficiencies, and von Willebrand studies. If these are normal, then the second tier of diagnostic work-up should include platelet function assays via platelet function analyzer and platelet aggregation assays. Abnormalities of the platelet function studies is enough for a diagnosis of QPD. However, flow cytometry may be used to delineate the rarer Glanzmann's thrombasthesnia and Bernard-Soulier disease, both subtypes of QPD. Electron microscopy can also be used, if available, to diagnose the subtypes of QPD such as gray platelet syndrome, alpha granule deficiency, etc.

Q2	What is the treatment of choice for QPD?

Therapy of choice for QPD depends on the specific cause of bleeding. In this patient's case, her menorrhagia was well-controlled with antifibrinolytics such as aminocaproic acid/tranexemic acid. At our center, we typically recommend patients take the antifibrinolytics for the duration of menses+2 additional days to ensure that bleeding does not recur. Oral contraception to regulate menses is another option for menorrhagia. The antifibrinolytics would also be the drug of choice for any routine dental procedures as well as epistaxis.

Q3	What is the role of DDAVP?

DDAVP is also an option, but not all patients with QPD respond to DDAVP. As such, in our center, we typically administer a DDAVP challenge to determine the response to this drug prior to prescribing it. In the event a patient is taken to surgery, again depends on the type of surgery. In more invasive procedures such as wisdom teeth extraction, or any other general surgery, the transfusion of platelets is warranted. DDAVP is also an option, provided, as above, they are known to respond to this drug. For refractory bleeding, recombinant factor VIIa is also an option to achieve emergent hemostasis.

This patient eventually required tonsillectomy for frequent pharyngitis. She was known to be a nonresponder to DDAVP. Pre-operatively, she received a dose of apheresis single donor platelet transfusion and had no bleeding complications.

Reference

Poon MC, D'Oiron R, Von Depka M, *et al.* (2004) Prophylactic and therapeutic recombinant factor VIIa administration to patients with Glanzmann thrombasthenia: results of an international survey. *J Thromb Haemost* **2**: 1096–1103.

PART IV

Acquired Bleeding Disorders

CASE STUDY 44

Acquired FVIII Inhibitor and B Cell Neoplasm

Alice D. Ma

Division of Hematology/Oncology, University of North Carolina, Chapel Hill, NC, USA

A 77-year-old woman with diabetes and psoriasis presented with new onset right leg swelling and painful "knots" under her skin. Duplex ultrasound and Doppler studies were negative for deep vein thrombosis. Further evaluation revealed a normal PT of 14 sec, and prolonged aPTT of 90 sec (25–32). 1:1 mixing studies showed 38 sec immediately, and 63 sec at 1 h incubation at 37 °C. Activity levels of FIX and XI were normal. FVIII activity level was <1%. Bethesda titer was 9 BU. Overnight, her hemoglobin fell by 1.4 g/dL, and the leg swelling worsened.

Q	How should the patient best be treated at this point?

The patient has developed an acquired inhibitor to FVIII – a rare autoimmune condition. Proper treatment requires a two-pronged approach. Bleeding cessation must be achieved with appropriate factor therapy, and immunosuppression should be started to eradicate the inhibitory autoantibody. Recombinant-activated FVII is approved in the USA for this indication at a dose of 70–90 mcg/kg IV given every 2 h until bleeding cessation. aPCCs can also be used at a dose of 75–100 units/kg every 8–12 h. Bypassing agents must be used when the Bethesda titer is above 5, the level at which FVIII concentrates are unlikely to show a therapeutic benefit. Our center has reported the use of single agent rituximab for the treatment of patients like this one. We have found that those with Bethesda titers less than 150 BU may need no further immunosuppression than 4 weekly doses of rituximab, 375 mg/m^2.

Hemophilia and Hemostasis: A Case-Based Approach to Management, Second Edition.
Edited by Alice D. Ma, Harold R. Roberts, Miguel A. Escobar.
© 2013 John Wiley & Sons, Ltd. Published 2013 by John Wiley & Sons, Ltd.

This patient was subsequently found to have abnormal lymphoid cells in her peripheral smear. Flow cytometry showed a monoclonal B cell population negative for CD5 and CD10. The peripheral lymphocyte count was 1.4×10^9/L. A bone marrow aspiration and biopsy was performed under coverage with rVIIa. It returned showing 2% involvement by a low grade B cell neoplasm. Notably, the patient had a CBC showing abnormal lymphoid cells 2–3 years prior to presentation. She had no B symptoms. CT scan showed no adenopathy in her chest, abdomen, or pelvis. There was a 4-cm liver lesion suspicious for involvement with lymphoma that had been unchanged for 5 years.

We therefore began therapy with rituximab, with hope that this agent would treat both the B cell process as well as the acquired hemophilia.

In general, our practice is not to do an extensive malignancy evaluation in patients who present with acquired hemophilia. Even if the patient presents with GI or GU bleeding, we try to not perform invasive procedures such as cystoscopy with bladder biopsy or colonoscopy with polyp removal. Rarely does this return positive for malignancy, and can lead to more severe bleeding. Any evaluation should wait until the inhibitor has resolved.

References

Boles JC, Key NS, Kasthuri R, Ma AD (2011) Single-center experience with rituximab as first-line immunosuppression for acquired hemophilia. *J Thromb Haemost* **9**(7): 1429–1431.

Collins PW (2011) Management of acquired haemophilia A. *J Thromb Haemost* **9**(Suppl 1): 226–235.

Ma AD, Carrizosa D (2006) *Acquired Factor VIII Inhibitors: Pathophysiology and Treatment.* ASH Educ. Book, pp. 432–437.

CASE STUDY 45

FVIII Inhibitor and Lupus Inhibitor

Alice D. Ma

Division of Hematology/Oncology, University of North Carolina, Chapel Hill, NC, USA

A 65-year-old man with prior history of a known lupus inhibitor presented with new-onset bleeding. He had a large hematoma in his left thigh and received rVIIa prior to transfer.

- Lupus PTT was elevated at 116 sec with positive platelet neutralization. The DRVVT was normal.
- Factor assays are shown in Table 45.1.

Q	We suspect the patient has developed a specific factor inhibitor in addition to his lupus inhibitor. How can we show this?

The following steps can be taken to show specificity of an inhibitor to a particular clotting factor. It is designed to pick up very weak inhibitors.

1 Dilute patient plasma sequentially with buffer, then use these diluted samples in mixing studies with normal plasma.
2 Perform PTT mixing studies.
3 Determine dilution at which PTT mixing studies just start to prolong.
4 Use this dilution and repeat clotting factor activity assays on the patient's plasma and control plasma

We diluted the patient and control plasma at 1:64, which was the point at which the PTT mix began to prolong with the buffer. After incubation, we repeated assays for factors previously found to be low. The results are shown in Table 45.2.

Hemophilia and Hemostasis: A Case-Based Approach to Management, Second Edition. Edited by Alice D. Ma, Harold R. Roberts, Miguel A. Escobar.
© 2013 John Wiley & Sons, Ltd. Published 2013 by John Wiley & Sons, Ltd.

Table 45.1 Activity levels for the various clotting factors. Multiple clotting factors are below normal limits, including FVIII, FIX, FXI, and FXII.

Factor	Activity level
II	112%
V	92%
VII	63%
VIII	20%
IX	16%
X	94%
XI	8%
XII	<7%

Table 45.2 Activity levels in control and patient plasma for the various clotting factors after dilution with buffer at 1:64. At this point, the only clotting factor out of the normal range is now FVIII. The effect of the non-specific inhibitor has been diluted away, and the only low factor activity is the factor against which there is a specific inhibitor.

Factor	Control	Patient
FVIII	48%	1%
FIX	67%	59%
FXI	43%	37%

This was consistent with acquired FVIII inhibitor in addition to the pre-existing lupus inhibitor.

CASE STUDY 46

Acquired von Willebrand Disease

Alice D. Ma

Division of Hematology/Oncology, University of North Carolina, Chapel Hill, NC, USA

A 72-year-old man presented from another hospital for management of lower GI bleeding and "Factor IX inhibitor." Per the referring physician, the patient was diagnosed as having a Factor IX inhibitor when he began having increasingly severe GI bleeding 18 months ago. The patient has had numerous AVMs in the upper and lower GI system, requiring cauterization and transfusion. The patient began therapy with cyclophosphamide and prednisone 15 months prior. He underwent colonoscopy with polypectomy 2 months ago. He was readmitted twice, requiring cauterization and transfusions, most recently 3–4 days prior to transfer to our institution. The patient was treated with FFP, repeat cauterization, and a single dose of rVIIa (2.4 mg=25 mcg/kg).

Laboratory records from referring doctor's office from 18 months ago show a FVIII activity of 52.6%. The FIX activity level was reported as 277%, with notice made of a "strong inhibitor present" are shown in Table 46.1.

Q1	Does the patient have an inhibitor to FIX?

Of course not. The diagnosis of a FIX inhibitor reflects misunderstanding of the term "strong inhibitor present." This terminology refers to the fact that a substance is interfering with the assay. The fact that the FIX activity was measured at 277% of normal rules out a function-blocking antibody to FIX.

History obtained at our center includes a long history of abnormal mucocutaneous bleeding. He bled abnormally from polypectomy 7 years

Hemophilia and Hemostasis: A Case-Based Approach to Management, Second Edition.
Edited by Alice D. Ma, Harold R. Roberts, Miguel A. Escobar.
© 2013 John Wiley & Sons, Ltd. Published 2013 by John Wiley & Sons, Ltd.

Table 46.1 Results for coagulation testing, along with normal values.

		Normal range
PT	12.9 sec	11–14
aPTT	73.4 sec	22.6–32.4
aPTT mix (immediate)	51 sec	–
aPTT mix (incubated)	57.4 sec	–

ago – required cauterization and transfusion. Abnormal bleeding with cuts and shaving, positive gum bleeding, nose bleeds. There is no family history of bleeding. On presentation, the patient was taking cyclophosphamide, pantoprazole, glimepiride, and pioglitazone. Physical examination showed a slightly cushingoid man, bad dentition, benign abdomen, no petechiae, and some bruising at line sites. The patient's labs were notable for a normal PT, a prolonged aPTT which failed to correct with 1:1 mixing. Additionally, there was no re-prolongation with incubation of the 1:1 mix (Table 46.1).

Q2	What is the differential diagnosis for the patient's laboratory values?

The patient has an isolated prolonged aPTT which fails to correct with mixing 1:1 with normal plasma. The aPTT does not prolong further with incubation at 37 °C. This pattern is consistent with either a lupus inhibitor or an acquired FVIII inhibitor. Factor levels were subsequently obtained, as shown in Table 46.2.

Lupus inhibitor testing was also obtained, results of which are shown in Table 46.3.

Q3	How would you interpret the above results?

The patient clearly has a phospholipid-dependent, or "lupus" inhibitor. There are nonlinear patterns to the assays of the factors that depend on the aPTT. However, the patient also has a very low FVIII activity level and a long history of mucocutaneous bleeding. An acquired FVIII inhibitor is still in the picture, but there is another acquired hemorrhagic disorder that now comes to mind.

Table 46.2 Activity levels for the various clotting factors.

		Normal range
Factor II	84%	78–122
Factor V	>162%**	59–100
Factor VII	69%	51–163
Factor VIII	<1%	61–158
Factor IX	>52%**	57–136
Factor X	75%	51–146
Factor XI	>52%**	49–100
Factor XII	>48%**	46–126

**inhibitory effect noted. Nonlinear assay

Table 46.3 Results of lupus inhibitor testing.

		Normal range
DRVVT	66.2 sec	0–35.2
DRVVT confirm	37 sec	–
DRVVT conf ratio	1.79	0.00–1.14
Lupus aPTT	105.9 sec	30–51.2
HPN w/o PL	110 sec	–
HPN w/ PL	75 sec	–
HPN Difference	35	–13.3 – 7.9

Table 46.4 Results for the PFA-100 closure times, along with normal values.

Collagen/epinephrine	>230 sec	84–178
Collagen/ADP	>228 sec	60–107

More labs were obtained, as indicated in Table 46.4 and Table 46.5. Notably, the hemoglobin was normal at 13 g/dL.

Q4	Is there another laboratory study you'd like to order?

Table 46.5 Results of VWF antigen and activity testing.

VWF Antigen	18%	50–199
VWF Activity	<9%	50–199

Table 46.6 Quantitative immuglobulin levels results.

	Patient's results	normal
IGG,SERUM	873MG/DL	525–1,650
IGM,SERUM	182MG/DL	25–210
IGA,SERUM	265MG/DL	40–390

An SPEP and immunofixation were obtained because of the consideration of acquired von Willebrand disease as a diagnosis. Quantitative immunoglobulin levels are shown in Table 46.6.

SPEP showed

The immunofixation of the serum showed a monoclonal component. Serum protein electrophoresis and immunofixation showed a monoclonal IgM kappa as well as free kappa light chains. The concentration of the IgM kappa was 0.4 g/dL.

Q5	Now what is the diagnosis?

The patient has a lupus inhibitor. He also has acquired VWD associated with a monoclonal gammopathy. Patients like this can be treated effectively with intravenous immunoglobulin infusions for bleeding episodes or prior to invasive procedures.

Q6	What are other causes of acquired VWD?

An acquired type 2 VWD can be seen in high shear cardiac lesions such as aortic stenosis or a ventricular septal defect. This is increasingly being seen in conjunction with left ventricular assist devices. This disorder also leads to chronic GI bleeding due to GI AVMs. An acquired type 2 VWD is also seen in myeloproliferative disorders with high platelet counts (usually >1,500 × 10⁹/L).

Severe hypothyroidism can lead to a type 1 VWD due to decreased synthesis of VWF. Pediatric patients with Wilm's tumors or other solid tumors can also present with acquired VWD.

Reference

Shetty S, Kasatkar P, Ghosh K (2011) Pathophysiology of acquired von Willebrand disease: a concise review. *Eur J Haematol* **87**: 99–106.

A Woman with Bleeding Gums

Alice D. Ma

Division of Hematology/Oncology, University of North Carolina, Chapel Hill, NC, USA

A 55-year-old woman presented with 1 month history of progressive leg swelling and fatigue. On evaluation, she was found to be in congestive heart failure. She had 4+ edema to her thighs and had nephrotic range-proteinuria. Hematology was consulted because of her complaint of spontaneous gum bleeding and bruising. Her PT and aPTT were both prolonged. CBC showed only mild anemia and rouleaux formation.

Q	What is (are) the most likely diagnosis (diagnoses)?

The nephrotic range proteinuria, CHF, and mild anemia suggest a diagnosis of amyloidosis. Patients with amyloidosis may have acquired FX deficiency due to the amyloid protein binding and removing the FX from the circulation. Thus, this disorder is a true acquired FX deficiency, rather than an autoantibody to the clotting factor, such as is seen in acquired hemophilia.

It has been reported that individuals with acquired FX deficiency due to amyloidosis may benefit from splenectomy if they have splenomegaly, thus removing a large reservoir of the amyloid protein and abrogating the coagulopathy.

The patients who are bleeding may require FX replacement with Prothrombin complex concentrates (PCCs). PCCs currently available in the United States include Bebulin VH (Baxter) and Profilnine SD (Grifols). These products both vary in their factor content, with Bebulin showing X>II>IX>VII and Profilnine having II>IX=X>VII, and both are virally

---

Hemophilia and Hemostasis: A Case-Based Approach to Management, Second Edition.
Edited by Alice D. Ma, Harold R. Roberts, Miguel A. Escobar.
© 2013 John Wiley & Sons, Ltd. Published 2013 by John Wiley & Sons, Ltd.

inactivated plasma-derived products. Remember that the half-life of factor X in these patients may be much lower than the 40–45 h seen in normal individuals.

Reference

Thompson CA, Kyle R, Gertz M, *et al.* (2010) Systemic AL amyloidosis with acquired factor X deficiency: a study of perioperative bleeding risk and treatment outcomes in 60 patients. *Am J Hematol* **85**: 171–173.

CASE STUDY 48

Bleeding after Cardiac Surgery

Alice D. Ma

Division of Hematology/Oncology, University of North Carolina, Chapel Hill, NC, USA

A 72-year-old man underwent aortic valve replacement and redo coronary artery bypass grafting at a local hospital. The patient had an uncomplicated recovery, was stabilized on warfarin, and was discharged to home on post-operative day 10. Three days later, the patient presented with chest pain and dyspnea and was found to have left-sided hemothorax, with a 2 g decrease in hemoglobin.

Initial labs tests showed PT 47 sec and aPTT 140 sec. Patient was given FFP, vitamin K, pRBCs, and had a chest tube placed. He remained stable for several days, during which the following laboratory studies were obtained:

- PT: 47 sec (12–14 sec)
- PT mix: 43 sec
- aPTT: 149 sec (25–33 sec)
- aPTT mix: 132 sec
- Lupus inhibitor was said to be "positive"
- Factor levels: II<1%, V<3 %, VII<3% VIII<2%, IX 10%, X<3%, XI<5%, XII<3%

The patient's local hematologist called for help from the HTC. The patient remained stable for several days without bleeding. Plasma was frozen and sent on dry ice to the coagulation laboratory at our center. On the day the sample was received, the patient developed a bloody pericardial effusion with tamponade and began bleeding from his chest tube. He had several cardiac arrests and was hypotensive on pressor agents in the ICU. He received 18 units of PRBC, 20 units of cryoprecipitate, and 24 units of FFP without halt in bleeding.

Hemophilia and Hemostasis: A Case-Based Approach to Management, Second Edition.
Edited by Alice D. Ma, Harold R. Roberts, Miguel A. Escobar.
© 2013 John Wiley & Sons, Ltd. Published 2013 by John Wiley & Sons, Ltd.

Table 48.1 Lupus inhibitor results showed no phospholipid-dependent inhibitor.

		Normal range
DRVVT	>150 sec	0–35.2 sec
DRVVT+phospholipid	>150 sec	
DRVVT ratio	Unable to calculate	
Lupus aPTT	>150 sec	0–35.2 sec
HPN w/o PL	188.2 sec	
HPN w/ PL	183 sec	
HPN Difference	5.2	−13.2–7.9

Table 48.2 Factor levels.

		Normal range
II	>53% **	78–122
V	<1%	59–100
VII	2%	51–163
VIII	>400% **	61–158
IX	>108% **	57–136
X	>71% **	51–146
XI	>51% **	49–100

**=nonlinear assay. Inhibitory pattern seen

Q1	What are some questions to be asked in this case?

I'd like to know if there was a nonlinear pattern observed for any of the assays of clotting factor activity. I'd also like to know the results of the lupus inhibitor assay (Table 48.1).

Blood was sent to our reference laboratory, and we obtained quite discrepant results for the clotting factor and lupus inhibitor assays (Table 48.2).

Q2	What explains the discrepancies between the clotting factor and lupus inhibitor assays between the different laboratories?

First, this community hospital laboratory performed only a DRVVT. Since it was prolonged, they interpreted this as consistent with a positive lupus inhibitor assay. This is not correct. While lupus inhibitors can prolong the DRVVT, lupus inhibitors are only one such cause. In fact, deficiencies of clotting factors X, V, II, and fibrinogen can also lead to a prolonged DRVVT. In order to diagnose a lupus inhibitor, the DRVVT must shorten by a certain amount upon addition of exogenous phospholipid. This step is required to diagnose a "phospholipid-dependent" inhibitor.

Next, the outside laboratory only performed factor assays at one single dilution point. Thus they missed the fact that the assays for factors II, VIII, IX, X, and XI showed progressive increase in the apparent factor activity with deeper dilutions of the patient sample. This is what is meant by a "nonlinear assay pattern." Serial dilutions of the patient's plasma must be performed in order to see or exclude such an inhibitory effect which is seen when there is a nonspecific inhibitor in the sample. Notably, the FV assay was low and did not show an inhibitory pattern, since the level never rose with serial dilutions – it just stayed low.

Q3	What does the patient have, and how should he be treated?

The patient has an acquired factor V inhibitor. These were most commonly seen after "redo" vascular or cardiac surgeries. The thrombin glue used in such procedures was formerly bovine thrombin which was contaminated with a small amount of bovine FV. Antibodies to bovine FV can cross-react and inhibit human FV, thus prolonging the PT and aPTT. Bovine thrombin glue is used in fewer centers, and the incidence of this disorder is declining. A recent review suggested that this disorder is more frequently associated with autoimmune conditions and cancer now.

Patients with acquired FV antibodies are typically asymptomatic, but occasionally, they can suffer hemorrhagic complications. The inhibitors are also typically transient, but treatment may be required to treat bleeding. Bleeding can be treated with transfusion of platelets, which carry 20% of the body's FV. The platelet FV is relatively resistant to inhibition by antibodies. Inhibitor eradication may require corticosteroids, IVIg, or plasma exchange.

Reference

Franchini M, Lippi G (2011) Acquired factor V inhibitors: a systematic review. *J Thromb Thrombolysis* **31**(4): 449–457.

CASE STUDY 49

Bleeding in a Dialysis Patient

Alice D. Ma

Division of Hematology/Oncology, University of North Carolina, Chapel Hill, NC, USA

A 55-year-old man with end stage renal disease on hemodialysis for the past 13 months, presented with profound gum bleeding and bleeding around the site of his dialysis catheter. He had worsening bleeding over the past 2 weeks, despite withholding heparin from his dialysate. He had no personal or family history of abnormal bleeding, and did not bleed with his prior kidney biopsy or with placement of his dialysis catheter 16 months ago. PMHx showed only severe hypertension and poor dentition. A physical examination showed raw, inflamed gums with small arterial bleeding from several sites. He had a raised rash around the base of his hair shafts on his legs and abdomen.

PT and aPTT were normal. VWF antigen and activity levels were markedly elevated. Platelet count was normal. TCT was normal.

Q	What is the likely diagnosis?

Because of the gingival inflammation and bleeding, as well as the perifollicular rash, a vitamin C level was sent and returned as undetectable. He was treated with high doses of vitamin C. In retrospect, he had been nonadherent with his nephrovites. He lived alone and only ate frozen burritos. He ate no fruit or vegetable.

Scurvy is unfortunately more common in the patients undergoing renal replacement therapy, since hemodialysis removes a significant amount of vitamin C. Additionally, most foods high in vitamin C are also high in potassium, and dialysis patients are warned away from these foods.

Hemophilia and Hemostasis: A Case-Based Approach to Management, Second Edition.
Edited by Alice D. Ma, Harold R. Roberts, Miguel A. Escobar.
© 2013 John Wiley & Sons, Ltd. Published 2013 by John Wiley & Sons, Ltd.

Supplementation is recommended, and nephrovites have vitamin C sufficient to replace losses during dialysis.

Reference

Handelman GJ (2007) Vitamin C deficiency in dialysis patients – Are we perceiving the tip of an iceberg? *Nephrol Dial Transplant* **22**(2): 328–331.

CASE STUDY 50

A Woman with Anemia and Hematuria

Alice D. Ma

Division of Hematology/Oncology, University of North Carolina, Chapel Hill, NC, USA

A 60-year-old African- American woman presented with new onset painless hematuria and fatigue of 2 weeks duration. She had well controlled hypertension, a history of fibroids, and had undergone hysterectomy at age 45 without difficulty. She had 4 children, all alive and well, and their deliveries were uncomplicated.

A physical examination was unremarkable. She had no flank tenderness or costovertebral pain. Laboratory studies showed anemia with Hgb 8 g/dL, normal WBC and platelets. Serum chemistries showed a Cre of 1.8 mg/dL and a decreased anion gap. Serum protein electrophoresis and immunofixation showed a monoclonal IgG lambda of 4 g/dL. Urinalysis showed red cells with no casts or crystals. The serum calcium was normal. Skeletal survey showed a small lytic lesion in the right 7th anterior rib and in the calvarium. PT was elevated at 14 sec (12–13.5) and aPTT was elevated at 95 sec (25–35). Mixing study failed to correct the aPTT, which remained elevated at 55 sec.

Q1	How should this patient be evaluated further?

The patient underwent bone marrow aspirate showing 30% monoclonal plasma cells. Cytogenetics were normal. The patient had profuse prolonged bleeding from her biopsy site and dropped her hemoglobin by 4 g/dL. The patient underwent further coagulation testing. All clotting factors were within normal limits, but all PTT-based assays showed a nonlinear pattern. The TCT was markedly prolonged at 30 sec (8–12). The reptilase time was

---

Hemophilia and Hemostasis: A Case-Based Approach to Management, Second Edition.
Edited by Alice D. Ma, Harold R. Roberts, Miguel A. Escobar.
© 2013 John Wiley & Sons, Ltd. Published 2013 by John Wiley & Sons, Ltd.

normal. Incubation with hepasorb corrected the aPTT, confirming the presence of a heparin-like substance.

Q2	How should this patient be treated?

A trial of protamine was given for 5 days, with prompt resolution of bleeding. She was started on systemic chemotherapy, and her bleeding never recurred.

Bleeding can occur in plasma cell dyscrasias via a number of mechanisms. The paraprotein may interfere with fibrinogen polymerization, in which case both the TT and the RT should be prolonged. Acquired deficiencies of PAI-1 and alpha-2 antiplasmin have also been reported, along with acquired FX deficiency. Additionally, a nonspecific acquired platelet dysfunction can occur.

Reference

Coppola A, Tufano A, Di Capua M, Franchini M (2011) Bleeding and thrombosis in multiple myeloma and related plasma cell disorders. *Semin Thromb Hemost* **37**(8): 929–945.

CASE STUDY 51

Scalp Bleeding in an Older Gentleman

Alice D. Ma

Division of Hematology/Oncology, University of North Carolina, Chapel Hill, NC, USA

An 83-year-old man presented for evaluation of persistent abnormal bleeding. The patient reported that his symptoms began 4 months prior to this evaluation. While installing a dishwasher, he hit his head on the underside of the cabinet. He developed a small scalp lesion at that time, which stopped bleeding normally. He reported no problems for approximately 6 weeks, after which time the lesion opened up and began to rebleed. When the bleeding did not subside, he presented to the Emergency Department in August (5 weeks prior to evaluation) and had sutures placed.

At the time of surgical follow-up, he had developed a large scalp hematoma such that the surgeon felt suture removal was unwise. He was referred to an outside hematologist who noted a normal PT and aPTT, normal VWF levels, but markedly abnormal PFA-100®.

The patient underwent surgical debridement, with complications of significant bleeding during this procedure, despite pretreatment with DDAVP and transfusion of platelets. The surgeon was quite voluble in his descriptions of the bleeding. Apparently, the patient's scalp bled with the slightest touch and would not stop. Since then, he has had daily significant bleeding requiring pressure dressings.

His personal history of bleeding is otherwise negative, despite having undergone multiple surgical procedures, including removal of brain absesses×2, hernia repair×2, dental surgery, and a cardiac catheterization. The patient takes no aspirin or nonsteroidal anti-inflammatory agents. There is no family history of bleeding. Medications included carbamazepine, lovastatin, ramipril, B12.

Hemophilia and Hemostasis: A Case-Based Approach to Management, Second Edition.
Edited by Alice D. Ma, Harold R. Roberts, Miguel A. Escobar.
© 2013 John Wiley & Sons, Ltd. Published 2013 by John Wiley & Sons, Ltd.

Physical examination revealed a slight older man wearing a pressure dressing on his scalp which he declined to remove. He had no petechiae or ecchymoses otherwise.

The patient had closure times of 300s in both the collagen/epinephrine and collagen/ADP cartridges of the PFA-100®. VWF activity and antigen were 85% and 94% of normal, respectively. The alpha-2 antiplasmin activity was 90% of normal. The PT and aPTT were normal. Platelet aggregation studies showed normal aggregation in response to thrombin, collagen, arachidonic acid, and 20 micromolar ADP. There was a decreased response to 2, 4, and 5 micromolar ADP, as well as to epinephrine. Normal agglutination to ristocetin was seen.

Q	What are some potential explanations for this patient's bleeding?

The patient has a mild defect in platelet aggregation associated with a profound prolongation of the PFA-100®. However, this should have been corrected with the transfusion of platelets. We suspected underlying tissue fragility and recommended careful surgical excision.

Upon examination of the scalp, the tissue appeared quite abnormally vascular, and biopsies revealed the presence of angiosarcoma, felt to be 11 cm in diameter. He underwent wide excision and split thickness skin grafting, but suffered near-immediate recurrence of disease within several weeks. Neither radiation nor chemotherapy was felt to offer any significant palliation or increase in disease-free survival.

Angiosarcomas – These are rare hemorrhagic tumors that can present with recurrent unexplained bleeding. Any patient with recurrent bleeding in the same anatomic location who has no personal or family history of a bleeding diathesis should have this diagnosis considered.

Reference

Bhatia S, Thomas CV, Hodder SC (2009) An interesting case – not an innocent haematoma! *Br J Oral Maxillofac Surg* **47**(6): 499.

CASE STUDY 52
Hyperfibrinolysis

Miguel A. Escobar[1,2,3] *and Anas Alrwas*[1]
[1] Department of Internal Medicine
[2] Division of Hematology, University of Texas Health Science Center at Houston
[3] Gulf States Hemophilia and Thrombophilia Center, Houston, TX, USA

A 50-year-old Hispanic male with a history of androgen-independent prostate cancer and kidney stones was admitted to our hospital for new-onset bleeding diathesis. His prostate cancer was originally diagnosed 8 months ago at an outside facility when he presented with hematuria. A work-up showed a prostate-specific antigen (PSA) of 1,200 ng/mL, and bone marrow involvement. Metastases to the ribs, left shoulder, and pelvis were also evidenced by a bone scan. The patient initially responded to bicalutamide, leuprolide, and zoledronic acid; however, the disease progressed 4 months later with a rising PSA. His treatment was then changed to ketoconazole and prednisone. After 7 months of treatment, the patient began to notice bruising on his torso and lower extremities. He required admission to the hospital in two occasions for bleeding complications. The first admission was for hemarthrosis in his left knee. His fibrinogen level was low, and the PT and aPTT were elevated. He received cryoprecipitate for presumed disseminated intravascular coagulation (DIC) with a temporary increase in fibrinogen level. The most recent hospitalization was due to a significant amount of bleeding after a bone marrow biopsy and aspirate, in which the patient had severe bruising of his lower back that tracked down to his left leg (Figure 52.1). In another instance, an attempt to place an IV in the patient's arm at an outside hospital resulted in severe bleeding at the puncture site requiring a thrombin dressing application. Due to these complications, the patient was transferred to our teaching institution for further care of his prostate cancer and coagulopathy.

Hemophilia and Hemostasis: A Case-Based Approach to Management, Second Edition.
Edited by Alice D. Ma, Harold R. Roberts, Miguel A. Escobar.
© 2013 John Wiley & Sons, Ltd. Published 2013 by John Wiley & Sons, Ltd.

(a) (b)

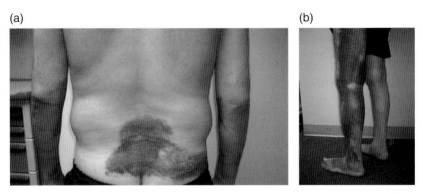

Figure 52.1 Hematoma formation after bone marrow biopsy. (a) Severe bruising of lower back and (b) down to patient's left leg.

At the time of presentation, the patient denied any hemoptysis, hematochezia, or hematuria. His past medical history was not significant for excessive bleeding or bruising.

His medications included ketoconazole, prednisone 5 mg twice a day; leuprolide every 3 months, hydrocodone and acetaminophen for pain. He reported no known drug allergies, and denied a history of smoking or alcohol abuse.

Laboratory data revealed a white blood cell count of 5.7 k/UL. Hemoglobin 7.8 g/DL, hematocrit 22.8%, and platelet count of 78,000 k/UL. PT was 15.9 sec (normal range 10.6–13.3 sec) that corrected with a 1:1 mixing study. The PTT was 42 sec (normal range 22.6–35.7 sec), fibrinogen 91.0 mg/dL (normal range 244–559) and D-dimer was greater than 5,000 ng/mL. Haptoglobin, electrolytes, hepatic, and renal function were normal. Lactate dehydrogenase was elevated at 1,401 IU/L (normal range 313–618). Factor VIII activity was 96% with a ristocetin cofactor activity of 237%.

Studies for hyperfibrinolysis included a thromboelastography that showed a prolonged lysis time LY30=39.2% (normal range 0–8). The euglobulin lysis time was short (<1 h) as well as the alpha-2-antiplasmin 57 units/dL (86–131).

Q	What is the diagnosis and how should the patient be managed?

Based on the above information, the presumptive diagnosis was hyperfibrinolysis. He was started on a continuous infusion of heparin intravenously at 200 units/h, which resulted in an improvement of the fibrinogen level and platelet count. In addition, an antifibrinolytic (epsilon aminocaproic acid) was given by mouth. The dose of heparin was increased to 400 units/h with further improvement in the fibrinogen levels. Finally the patient was discharged on low molecular weight heparin twice a day and aminocaproic acid. For the carcinoma he was treated with diethylstilbestrol plus dexamethasone followed by weekly docetaxel.

The heparin and antifibrinolytic were discontinued after about 30 days when the carcinoma was under control and there was no further evidence of hyperfibrinolysis.

Discussion

The term "primary fibrinolysis" entails systemic activation of plasmin or direct degradation of fibrinogen in the absence of disseminated intravascular coagulation (DIC). Acquired abnormalities of the fibrinolytic system such as DIC, chronic liver disease, trauma, coagulation factor deficiencies, plasminogen activators (i.e. streptokinase), major surgical procedures such as cardiopulmonary bypass, and heat stroke can cause markedly enhanced fibrinolytic activity, sometimes producing excessive bleeding, known as secondary hyperfibrinolysis. Hyperfibrinolysis has been reported with a number of malignancies such as prostate and gastric cancer, nonlymphoblastic, and promyelocytic leukemias.

The incidence of disseminated intravascular coagulation (DIC) in patients with metastatic prostate cancer is unknown because most patients are well compensated and without clinical manifestation of a coagulopathy. The occurrence of systemic fibrinolysis has been reported in patients with metastatic prostate cancer. It is due to excess production of urinary-type plasminogen activators by the malignant cells, and secondary reductions in alpha-2-antiplasmin.

Several investigators have provided experimental evidence that support the role of proteases such as urokinase plasminogen activator (uPA) in determining the invasive potential of prostate cancer. The uPA system seems to play an important role in promoting metastasis and angiogenesis. The inactive precursor of the serine protease, urokinase-type plasminogen activator is activated by binding a specific membrane-bound or soluble cell surface receptor (urokinase-type plasminogen activator receptor [uPAR]), which accelerates the conversion of plasminogen into plasmin, a serine protease that degrades fibrin and causes fibrinolysis. Shariat et al. (2007), showed that, in patients with prostate cancer, urokinase-type plasminogen activator (uPA) and its soluble receptor (uPAR) both increased significantly in patients with aggressive disease.

In a case series by Okajima et al. (1994), 8 patients were found to have systemic fibrinogenolysis. Three of the patients had gastric cancer, 2 were diagnosed with metastatic prostatic cancer, 2 had acute promyelocytic leukemia, and 1 had abdominal aortic aneurysm. In the 2 patients with prostate cancer, the level of alpha 2-plasmin inhibitor gradually increased with the reduction of tumor size by treatment.

Treatment with chemotherapy or epsilon-aminocaproic acid has been reported to reverse the coagulopathy due to prostate cancer associated hyperfibrinolysis. Sallah *et al.* (2000) described resolution of the fibrinolytic process in 5 of 8 patients who had hormone-refractory prostate cancer with bleeding and laboratory evidence of primary hyperfibrinogenolysis, after one cycle of treatment with docetaxel. In another report, Cooper *et al.* (1992) describe a patient with DIC and soft tissue hemorrhage after a prostatic biopsy that was successfully treated with epsilon-aminocaproic acid and low-dose heparin, as demonstrated by his fibrinogen levels rapidly returning to normal after therapy.

References

Andreasen PA, Kjoller L, Christensen L, *et al.* (1997). The urokinase-type plasminogen activator system in cancer metastasis: A review. *Int J Cancer* **72**: 1–22.

Cooper DL, Sandler AB, Wilson LD, Duffy TP (1992) Disseminated intravascular coagulation and excessive fibrinolysis in a patient with metastatic prostate cancer: response to epsilon-aminocaproic acid. *Cancer* **70**(3): 656–658.

Okajima K, Kohno I, Soe G, *et al.* (1994) Direct evidence for systemic fibrinogenolysis in patients with acquired alpha 2-plasmin inhibitor deficiency. *Am J Hematol* **45**(1): 16–24.

Rabbani SA, Mazar AP (2001) The role of the plasminogen activation system in angiogenesis and metastasis. *Surg Oncol Clin North Am* **10**: 393–415.

Sallah S, Gagnon GA (2000) A reversion of primary hyperfibrinogenolysis in patients with hormone-refractory prostate cancer using docetaxel. *Cancer Invest* **18**(3): 191–196.

Schmitt M, Harbeck N, Thomssen C, *et al.* (1997) Clinical impact of the plasminogen activation system in tumor invasion and metastasis: prognostic relevance and target for therapy. *Thromb Haemost* **78**(1): 285–296.

Shariat SF, Roehrborn CG, McConnel JD, *et al.* (2007) Association of the circulating levels of the urokinase system of plasminogen activation with the presence of prostate cancer and invasion, progression, and metastasis. *J Clin Oncol* **25**(4): 349–355.

PART V

Thrombotic Disorders

CASE STUDY 53

Heparin-Induced Thrombocytopenia with Thrombosis

Miguel A. Escobar

Division of Hematology, University of Texas Health Science Center at Houston and Gulf States Hemophilia and Thrombophilia Center, Houston, TX, USA

A 67-year-old man underwent an uncomplicated total knee replacement and received low molecular weight heparin (enoxaparin) post-operatively at a dose of 40 mg SC daily. 14 days later, the patient developed infection of the knee and underwent operative washout. He was subsequently restarted on the same dose of enoxaparin and a few days later, he noticed erythema at the site of injection associated with pain. This site later became necrotic (Figure 53.1). Nineteen days after the TKR, the patient developed an ischemic foot with evidence of a popliteal artery thrombosis by arteriogram (Figure 53.2). The ELISA test for heparin-induced thrombocytopenia (HIT) was positive, as was the serotonin release assay. His platelet count on admission was 75,000. He required amputation above the knee 5 days later.

Q	What should be the procedure if HIT is strongly suspected?

HIT is a serious and potentially fatal complication of heparin use that occurs in up to 5% of patients exposed to this medication. The use of low molecular weight heparin and shorter courses of exposure may be associated with a lower incidence of the disease. Other risk factors for the development of HIT include female gender, age > 40 years old, and surgical procedures – especially cardiovascular and orthopedic procedures. Thrombosis is a common complication of HIT seen in up to 50% of patients. Although venous thrombosis accounts for the majority of cases, limb ischemia can affect approximately 5–15% of patients, requiring amputation. In heparin-naïve patients, thrombocytopenia usually occurs between

Hemophilia and Hemostasis: A Case-Based Approach to Management, Second Edition.
Edited by Alice D. Ma, Harold R. Roberts, Miguel A. Escobar.
© 2013 John Wiley & Sons, Ltd. Published 2013 by John Wiley & Sons, Ltd.

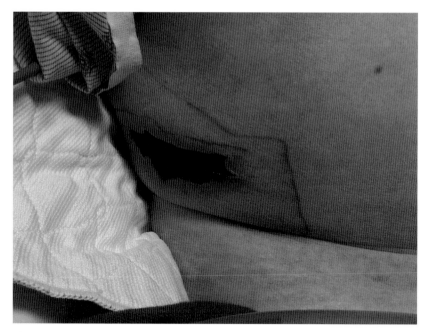

Figure 53.1 Skin necrosis at the site of enoxaparin injection.

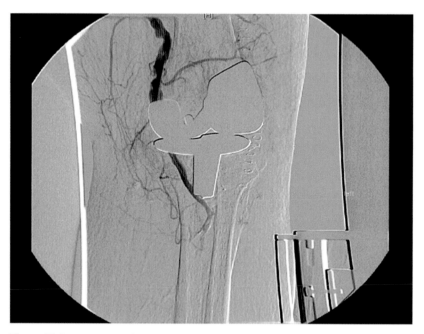

Figure 53.2 Arteriogram showing complete thrombosis of the popliteal artery.

the 5th and 11th day of exposure, with platelet counts dropping by at least 50% of baseline. In patients with a previous exposure to heparin, as in the above case, thrombocytopenia and thrombosis can occur much earlier.

Heparin antibodies can be found by the use of different techniques: platelet factor 4/polyanion enzyme immunoassays are more readily available in general laboratories but lack specificity as compared to platelet activation assays (serotonin release assay and heparin-induced platelet activation assay).

When HIT is strongly suspected, heparin should be discontinued and an alternative anticoagulant started. Direct thrombin inhibitors or anti-Xa inhibitors are the drugs of choice. Anticoagulation with warfarin should not be started until the platelet count has normalized and should be overlapped with a parenteral anticoagulant for at least 5 days.

Reference

Cuker A, Cines DB (2012) How I treat heparin-induced thrombocytopenia (HIT). *Blood*; doi:10.1182/blood-2011-11-376293.

CASE STUDY 54

Heparin Skin Necrosis

Miguel A. Escobar

Division of Hematology, University of Texas Health Science Center at Houston and Gulf States
Hemophilia and Thrombophilia Center, Houston, TX, USA

A 55-year-old white male was admitted after a fall from a deer tree stand. He had fractures of tibias, right hand, and multiple ribs. He received enoxaparin 40 mg SC daily for DVT prophylaxis. On day 5 he started to experience pain and erythema on the site of injection. By day 6 he noticed the skin became darker with evidence of vesicles (Figure 54.1). His platelet count was 727,000 and the ELISA for heparin-induced thrombocytopenia (HIT) was highly positive. Hematology was consulted. Heparin was discontinued and the patient was started on fondaparinux 2.5 mg SC/day and transitioned to warfarin for 3 months. He had no evidence of thrombosis or thrombocytopenia. Levels of protein S and C were also normal.

Q	What is the management of heparin skin necrosis without thrombocytopenia?

Heparin-induced skin necrosis is a rare complication of heparin therapy. The lesions usually become apparent by day 5 to 11 following initiation of treatment. Some patients develop thrombocytopenia and thrombosis in association with IgG heparin-platelet factor 4 antibodies. Although these patients with isolated skin necrosis may not have clinical evidence of thrombosis, adrenal hemorrhagic infarction and microvascular thrombi within the necrotic skin lesion have been reported. Arterial thrombosis may also be associated with heparin-induced skin necrosis.

The early recognition of heparin sensitivity is important to avoid the complications of HIT. Although in this specific case the platelet count never decreased, the early discontinuation of heparin most likely reduced the

---

Hemophilia and Hemostasis: A Case-Based Approach to Management, Second Edition.
Edited by Alice D. Ma, Harold R. Roberts, Miguel A. Escobar.
© 2013 John Wiley & Sons, Ltd. Published 2013 by John Wiley & Sons, Ltd.

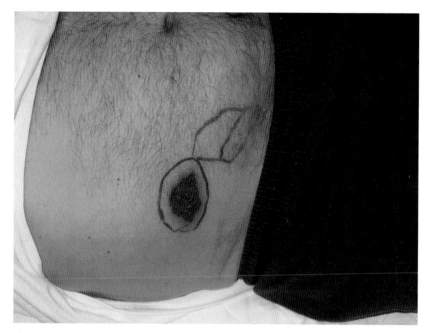

Figure 54.1 Skin lesion 6 days after injecting enoxaparin for DVT prophylaxis corresponding to heparin skin necrosis.

risks of thromboses. Prompt transition to alternative anticoagulants like thrombin inhibitors or Xa inhibitors is recommended.

References

Katsourakis A, *et al.* (2011) Low molecular weight heparin-induced skin necrosis: a case report. *Case Rep Med*: doi:10.1155/2011/857391.

Warkentin TE (1996) Heparin-induced skin lesions. *Br J Haematol* **92**: 494–497.

Warkentin TE, Roberts RS, Hirsh J, Kelton JG (2005) Heparin-induced skin lesions and other unusual sequelae of the heparin-induced thrombocytopenia syndrome: a nested cohort study. *Chest* **127**(5): 1857–1861.

CASE STUDY 55

Warfarin Skin Necrosis

Miguel A. Escobar

Division of Hematology, University of Texas Health Science Center at Houston and Gulf States
Hemophilia and Thrombophilia Center, Houston, TX, USA

A 44-year-old African-American female with a past history of lower extremity deep vein thrombosis and pulmonary embolism 10 years ago visited the emergency room complaining of tender skin lesions on both lower extremities (see Figure 55.1(a)). She had been on chronic anticoagulation with warfarin, but was having difficulty maintaining a therapeutic INR. On further questioning, she stated that, about 1 week ago, she visited her primary care physician, and her INR was only 1.7 on 5 mg of warfarin daily. He recommended increasing the warfarin dose to 10 mg a day and having a repeat INR in 1 week. Three days later, she started to have pain in her thighs where the skin lesions are located. On examination, the patient was in acute distress due to severe pain requiring intravenous morphine. She was afebrile and hemodynamically stable. Positive findings included two large erythematous lesions with vesicles on lateral aspect of both thighs and a hypopigmented scar on the right thigh. Her CBC and renal function were normal. The INR was 3.9 with a normal PTT and thrombin time. On further questioning, it was found that she had had a similar skin lesion 7 years ago, which corresponds to the scar in her leg (Figure 55.1(b)).

Q	What is the management of warfarin skin necrosis?

A clinical diagnosis of warfarin skin necrosis was made and enoxaparin was started at a dose of 1 mg/kg of body weight every 12 h. Vitamin K was given to reverse the effect of warfarin. Her skin lesions progressed to cutaneous necrosis with extensive ulceration that took over a year to heal.

Hemophilia and Hemostasis: A Case-Based Approach to Management, Second Edition.
Edited by Alice D. Ma, Harold R. Roberts, Miguel A. Escobar.
© 2013 John Wiley & Sons, Ltd. Published 2013 by John Wiley & Sons, Ltd.

(a)   (b)

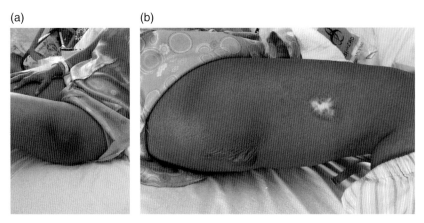

Figure 55.1 (a) Skin necrosis of thighs. (b) Evidence of a previous similar lesion 7 years ago.

Four weeks after being on low molecular weight heparin, thrombophilia studies revealed a total protein S of 40% (normal 58–146), free protein S of 52% (normal 62–146) with a normal protein C, homocysteine, antiphospholipid antibodies, antithrombin, and negative for factor V Leiden and prothrombin mutation.

Discussion

Warfarin-induced skin necrosis (WISN) is a rare disorder characterized by diffuse microthrombi within the dermal and subcutaneous vessels with endothelial damage resulting in necrosis. Warfarin produces a paradoxical hypercoagulable state by inhibiting the vitamin-K-dependent proteins like C and S. This prothrombotic state can be more pronounced in patients with a congenital deficiency of protein C and S. The majority of lesions appear in areas of abundant fatty tissue like the breasts, buttocks, and thighs. Initial treatment should be the use of a parenteral anticoagulant to avoid further thrombosis and the reversal of the vitamin K antagonist with vitamin K or fresh frozen plasma. Protein C concentrates can also be used for protein C deficiency. Extensive skin lesions may require debridement and skin grafting.

These patients can be put back on warfarin but that should be done slowly while on a parenteral anticoagulant. Incremental doses of warfarin should be small, and frequent monitoring is recommended.

References

Inayatullah S, Phadke G, Vilenski L, *et al.* (2010) Warfarin-induced skin necrosis. *Southern Med Assoc* **103**: 74–75.

Nazarian RM, Van Cott EM, Zembowicz A, Duncan LM (2009) Warfarin-induced skin necrosis. *J Am Acad Dermatol* **61**: 325–332.

CASE STUDY 56

Thoracic Outlet Syndrome

Tyler Buckner
Pediatric Hematology/Oncology, University of North Carolina School of Medicine,
Chapel Hill, NC, USA

A young female patient presented with persistent pain, swelling, and discoloration of the right arm. She had no other personal or family history of thrombosis. She was not on oral contraceptives. Obstruction of the right subclavian vein was suspected.

Q	What is the most helpful imaging study for this condition, and how should it be managed?

Deep-vein thrombosis (DVT) of the upper extremity is often secondary to another cause (intravenous catheters, cancer, surgery, or hormone-induced), but 20% of the time it is either idiopathic or due to abnormalities of the venous system at the costoclavicular junction. Compression of the subclavian vein by the clavicle, first rib, anterior scalene muscle, subclavius muscle, and/or costoclavicular ligament causes abnormalities of blood flow that may lead to thrombosis in the affected arm. This particular pathophysiologic process and its results are termed "the venous thoracic outlet syndrome".

The Paget–Schroetter syndrome, or subclavian vein effort thrombosis, is a related condition in which the subclavian vein undergoes repetitive compression during overhead arm extension, causing intimal injury and eventually perivenous fibrosis. The resulting stenosis is analogous to the narrowing seen in the venous thoracic outlet syndrome (which may also be present). The Paget–Schroetter syndrome is more commonly diagnosed in athletes or workers who repeatedly raise their arms over their heads (swimmers, weight-lifters, tennis players, painters, etc.).

Hemophilia and Hemostasis: A Case-Based Approach to Management, Second Edition.
Edited by Alice D. Ma, Harold R. Roberts, Miguel A. Escobar.
© 2013 John Wiley & Sons, Ltd. Published 2013 by John Wiley & Sons, Ltd.

In patients with DVT involving the upper extremity, diagnosis of venous thoracic outlet syndrome requires demonstration of stenosis of the subclavian vein at the costoclavicular junction. In patients with idiopathic or recurrent upper extremity DVT, CT or MR venography is often useful in examining the subclavian vein, though data regarding their accuracy in this condition are lacking. The gold standard test for venous thoracic outlet syndrome is contrast venography, often performed with the patient's arm raised to evaluate the full extent of subclavian vein compression.

Management of venous thoracic outlet syndrome and Paget–Schroetter syndrome is generally approached in a stepwise, risk-adapted fashion. Given the various therapeutic modalities involved, communication and cooperation between providers in multiple specialties is often required. Low-molecular-weight heparin or unfractionated heparin can be used for initial anticoagulation. The optimal duration for anticoagulation therapy is not known, but based on data for lower extremity DVT, 3 to 6 months of anticoagulation is generally recommended. Catheter-directed thrombolysis may be useful in patients with recent-onset, severe symptoms, if they are also at low risk of bleeding.

Patients who continue to have severe symptoms or recurrence of thrombosis despite anticoagulation and thrombolysis may benefit from mechanical catheter interventions, such as balloon angioplasty and thrombectomy. Stenting is not useful in venous thoracic outlet syndrome due to high rates of malfunction of these devices in the costoclavicular junction. Finally, surgical correction of the anatomical abnormality causing the subclavian vein compression can be undertaken in patients with persistent or recurrent symptoms. This procedure involves surgical decompression (by resecting the first rib and other involved structures) and sometimes subclavian vein reconstruction; in experienced centers, surgical outcomes are generally very good.

References

Kucher N (2011) Clinical practice. Deep-vein thrombosis of the upper extremities. *N Engl J Med* **364**(9): 861–869.

Melby SJ, Vedantham S, Narra VR, *et al.* (2008) Comprehensive surgical management of the competitive athlete with effort thrombosis of the subclavian vein (Paget–Schroetter syndrome). *J Vasc Surg* (official publication, the Society for Vascular Surgery [and] International Society for Cardiovascular Surgery, North American Chapter); issue **47**(4): 809–820; discussion 821.

CASE STUDY 57

Antithrombin Deficiency

Miguel A. Escobar

Division of Hematology, University of Texas Health Science Center at Houston and Gulf States Hemophilia and Thrombophilia Center, Houston, TX, USA

A 25-year-old female with a past medical history of congenital antithrombin (AT) deficiency, without previous thromboembolic events, visited our thrombophilia clinic because she was 6 weeks pregnant. She has a strong family history of venous thromboembolism (VTE) and antithrombin deficiency, which includes her mother, sister, and few cousins. Her AT level was 50% with an antigen of 17 IU/dL (normal >24). DNA analysis showed a missense mutation in exon 7 of the SERPINC1 gene, consistent with a diagnosis of type II antithrombin deficiency.

Q1	What is the management of antithrombin deficiency during pregnancy in this patient?

Although in this particular case there was no history of previous VTE, her risk for thrombosis during pregnancy was high. She was started on enoxaparin at 1 mg/kg SC every 12 h throughout the entire pregnancy. Anti-Xa levels were frequently monitored. Postpartum she remained on anticoagulation for 8 weeks.

Q2	Does replacement with AT concentrates play a role during pregnancy?

Antithrombin concentrates are indicated for the prevention of perioperative and peripartum thromboembolic events in hereditary antithrombin-deficient individuals. In the USA there are two commercial products

---

Hemophilia and Hemostasis: A Case-Based Approach to Management, Second Edition.
Edited by Alice D. Ma, Harold R. Roberts, Miguel A. Escobar.
© 2013 John Wiley & Sons, Ltd. Published 2013 by John Wiley & Sons, Ltd.

available: ATryn, a transgenic antithrombin, and Thrombate III, a purified human protein. Both products are for intravenous use. ATryn is used as a continuous infusion while Thrombate III is given in boluses. AT plasma levels should be monitored with the use of both products. The calculation of the dose is individualized based, on the baseline AT level and weight of the patient (see package insert of each product). Treatment should be initiated ~24 h before delivery and maintained for a few days postpartum. Anticoagulation can be restarted as soon as safe in the postpartum period and can be given concomitantly with the AT concentrates.

CASE STUDY 58

May–Thurner Syndrome

Trinh T. Nguyen[1] and Miguel A. Escobar[2]

[1] Division of Hematology, University of Texas Health Science Center at Houston
[2] Gulf States Hemophilia and Thrombophilia Center, Houston, TX, USA

A 13-year-old Hispanic girl presented to the ER with left lower thigh pain and swelling for 1 week. There were no provoking factors, including prolonged trips, birth control, or recent trauma. Work-up showed thrombus from the left popliteal to the left iliac vein. Hypercoagulable work-up was negative. MRI/MRV of the lower extremity to the pelvis showed occlusion of the left common iliac vein and external iliac vein from the level of the right common iliac artery crossing over the IVC/expected location of the left common femoral vein confluence.

Q1	What is the diagnostic suspicion for May–Thurner syndrome?

An unprovoked DVT in the location of the left iliofemoral region should prompt a work-up for the May–Thurner syndrome. The lifetime risk of recurrent thrombosis is upwards of 70%, while approximately 60% develop post-thrombotic syndrome characterized by edema, pain, dermatitis, and ulcers.

Q2	What is the management of this rare disease?

The mainstay of therapy for May–Thurner syndrome is vascular surgery intervention to administer thrombolytics followed by angioplasty +/− stenting (Figure 58.1). Anticoagulation serves as an adjunct.

Hemophilia and Hemostasis: A Case-Based Approach to Management, Second Edition.
Edited by Alice D. Ma, Harold R. Roberts, Miguel A. Escobar.
© 2013 John Wiley & Sons, Ltd. Published 2013 by John Wiley & Sons, Ltd.

(a)

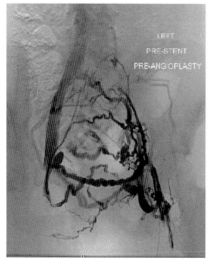 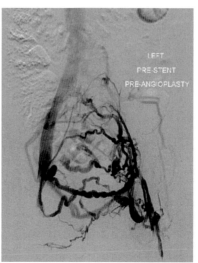

(b)

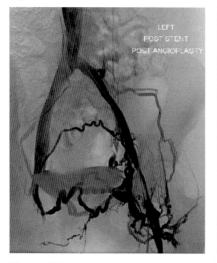 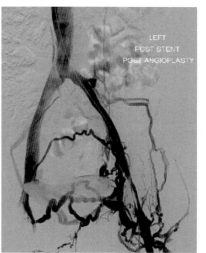

Figure 58.1 (a) Pre-stent; (b) post-stent.

References

Lamont JP, Pearl GJ, Patetsios P, *et al.* (2002) Prospective evaluation of endoluminal venous stents in the treatment of the May–Thurner syndrome. *Ann Vasc Surg* **16**(1): 61–64.

Moudgill N, Hager E, Gonsalves C, *et al.* (2009) May–Thurner syndrome: case report and review of the literature involving modern endovascular therapy. *Vascular* **17**(6): 330–335.

O'Sullivan GJ, Semba CP, Bittner CA, *et al.* (2000) Endovascular management of iliac vein compression (May–Thurner) syndrome. *J Vasc Interv Radiol* **11**(7): 823–836.

Patel NH, Stookey KR, Ketcham DB, Cragg AH (2000) Endovascular management of acute extensive iliofemoral deep venous thrombosis caused by May–Thurner syndrome. *J Vasc Interv Radiol* **11**(10):1297–1302.

CASE STUDY 59

Thrombosis in a Liver Transplant Patient

Alice D. Ma

Division of Hematology/Oncology, University of North Carolina, Chapel Hill, NC, USA

A 45-year-old man underwent an orthotopic liver transplant for liver failure due to nonaloholic steatotic hepatitis. The transplant procedure was uncomplicated, but 3–4 weeks after his transplant, he developed profound dyspnea and leg swelling and was diagnosed with a left DVT of the common femoral vein, as well as bilateral pulmonary emboli. He was anticoagulated with heparin and warfarin, but 1 month later, when his INR had fallen to 1.8, he developed a right leg DVT.

Personal and family history were negative for thromboembolic disease. He used neither alcohol nor tobacco. He did have diabetes mellitus and obesity.

Thrombophilia testing was performed. He was negative for factor V Leiden and the Prothrombin G20210 mutation. He had normal levels of antithrombin. Protein C and S were low, but he was on warfarin. Antiphospholipid antibody testing was negative. His FVIII activity level was 220% of normal.

Q	What other testing should be performed?

The patient underwent testing for APC resistance and had an APC resistance ratio of 0.45 (nl > 0.61). We hypothesized that the liver donor might have carried the gene for factor V Leiden. The DNA test was run on the recipient's own white cells, which were negative for the FVL mutation. However, the liver is the major source for FV, and this patient had acquired APC resistance due to a liver transplant from a donor with FVL. This could be proven if a biopsy of the transplanted liver were tested for the FVL mutation.

We recommended indefinite anticoagulation with more careful monitoring of INRs.

Hemophilia and Hemostasis: A Case-Based Approach to Management, Second Edition.
Edited by Alice D. Ma, Harold R. Roberts, Miguel A. Escobar.
© 2013 John Wiley & Sons, Ltd. Published 2013 by John Wiley & Sons, Ltd.

CASE STUDY 60

Combined Thrombophilia

Trinh T. Nguyen[1] and Miguel A. Escobar[2]
[1]Division of Hematology, University of Texas Health Science Center at Houston
[2]Gulf States Hemophilia and Thrombophilia Center, Houston, TX, USA

A 49-year-old man with history of hypertension, morbid obesity, and sleep apnea was admitted on May 2009 for a 2 week history of left arm pain. In the ER, he was noted to have decreased distal pulses of the left upper extremity. Work-up showed left axillary vein thrombosis, and he underwent thrombectomy 2 days later. Post-operatively, the thrombosis recurred and he required a repeat thrombectomy 9 days later. Anticoagulation was intiated with unfractionated heparin (UFH) for 2 weeks followed by Coumadin with a 3-day bridge with enoxaparin.

A hypercoagulable work-up revealed heterozygosity for the factor V Leiden mutation as well as the prothrombin gene mutation. He has been adherent to therapy with warfarin, with INR values consistently in the 2–3 range. He is also on baby aspirin 81 mg daily. He has persistent left arm pain with imaging showing severe cervical stenosis (C3–C4). Neurology recommended a trial of cervical epidural steroid injection.

Q1	Should this patient stop Coumadin and have the procedure or should he have bridging therapy?

Heterozygotes for factor V Leiden have a 5- to 7-fold risk of developing a DVT while a heterozygote for the prothrombin gene mutation has a 2- to 3-fold increased risk. Patients with combined heterozygosities, however, have a 20-fold risk of thrombosis. This patient has had recurrent LUE thrombosis requiring thrombectomy and, with his genetic predispositions to thrombosis, bridging therapy should be used prior to the procedure. If

---

Hemophilia and Hemostasis: A Case-Based Approach to Management, Second Edition.
Edited by Alice D. Ma, Harold R. Roberts, Miguel A. Escobar.
© 2013 John Wiley & Sons, Ltd. Published 2013 by John Wiley & Sons, Ltd.

he undergoes the steroid injections, according to ACCP 2012 guidelines, Coumadin should be discontinued 5 days prior to the procedure. Anticoagulation with low molecular weight heparin (LMWH) or unfractionated heparin (UFH) should commence. Economically, it is preferable to do outpatient LMWH injections rather than admitting the patient for IV UFH. Prior to the procedure, the dose of LMWH should be held at least 24 h. Moreover, the last dose before the LMWH is held pre-operatively is recommended to be 50% of the patient's regular dose. Post-operatively, since this is a minor procedure, LMWH should resume at least 24 h later. During bridging therapy, it is not recommended to routine check the anti-Xa level on a patient on LMWH.

Q2	Should this patient be off anticoagulation for any prolonged period of time?

Based on the ACCP 2012 guidelines, the aspirin should be discontinued 7–10 days prior to the procedure since he is at low risk for cardiovascular events. Post-operatively, when adequate hemostasis is ensured, he may restart aspirin.

The patient had two provoked DVTs requiring surgical thrombectomy. In this patient we would continue life-long anticoagulation as his risk factors are persistent, obesity, prior thromboses, and a high risk of recurrence.

References

Chamberlain AM, Folsom AR, Heckbert SR, *et al.* (2008) High-density lipoprotein cholesterol and venous thromboembolism in the Longitudinal Investigation of Thromboembolism Etiology (LITE). *Blood* **112**(7): 2675–2680.

Douketis JD, *et al.* (2012) Perioperative management of antithrombotic therapy: *Antithrombotic Therapy and Prevention of Thrombosis*. American College of Chest Physicians Evidence-Based Clinical Practice Guidelines (9th edn). *Chest* **141**(Suppl 2): 326–350.

Emmerich J, Rosendaal FR, Cattaneo M, *et al.* (2001) Combined effect of factor V Leiden and prothrombin 20210A on the risk of venous thromboembolism – pooled analysis of 8 case-control studies including 2310 cases and 3204 controls. Study group for pooled-analysis in venous thromboembolism. *Thromb Haemost* **86**(3): 809–816.

Rosendaal FR (2009) Genetics of venous thrombosis. *J Thromb Haemost* **7**(Suppl 1): 301–314.

Index

Note: Page references in *italics* refer to Figures; those in **bold** refer to Tables

Hemophilia and Hemostasis: A Case-Based Approach to Management, Second Edition.
Edited by Alice D. Ma, Harold R. Roberts, Miguel A. Escobar.
© 2013 John Wiley & Sons, Ltd. Published 2013 by John Wiley & Sons, Ltd.